Winning the Battle Against Prostate Cancer

GET THE TREATMENT THAT IS RIGHT FOR YOU

Winning the Battle Against Prostate Cancer

GET THE TREATMENT THAT IS RIGHT FOR YOU

Gerald Chodak, MD

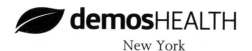
demosHEALTH

New York

ISBN 978-1-936303-03-8
Acquisitions Editor: Noreen Henson
Cover Design: Steve Pisano
Compositor: Absolute Service, Inc.
Printer: Hamilton Printing Company

Visit our website at www.demoshealth.com

Medical information provided by Demos Health, in the absence of a visit with a healthcare professional, must be considered as an educational service only. This book is not designed to replace a physician's independent judgment about the appropriateness or risks of a procedure or therapy for a given patient. Our purpose is to provide you with information that will help you make your own healthcare decisions.

The information and opinions provided here are believed to be accurate and sound, based on the best judgment available to the authors, editors, and publisher, but readers who fail to consult appropriate health authorities assume the risk of any injuries. The publisher is not responsible for errors or omissions. The editors and publisher welcome any reader to report to the publisher any discrepancies or inaccuracies noticed.

Library of Congress Cataloging-in-Publication Data
A catalog record for this book is available from the Library of Congress.

Special discounts on bulk quantities of Demos Health books are available to corporations, professional associations, pharmaceutical companies, health care organizations, and other qualifying groups. For details, please contact:

Special Sales Department
Demos Medical Publishing
11 W. 42nd Street
New York, NY 10036
Phone: 800–532–8663 or 212–683–0072
Fax: 212–941–7842
E-mail: rsantana@demosmedpub.com

Made in the United States of America
10 11 12 13   5 4 3 2 1

FOR ALL MEN WITH PROSTATE CANCER OR
YET TO BE DIAGNOSED WITH IT,
HOPING THOSE NEEDING TREATMENT GET CURED
AND ALL THE REST ARE NOT HARMED.

Contents

Foreword

Dr. Chodak has made a valuable contribution in writing this comprehensive book for the thousands of men battling prostate cancer. This book provides useful information in the fight against this under-recognized disease.

As America and the world ages, more men are at the age of risk from prostate cancer than ever before. This is the number one cancer diagnosed in men after skin cancer. It is diagnosed at a similar or higher level than breast cancer is in women. This fact is becoming more recognized and *Winning the Battle Against Prostate Cancer* provides information to millions of men, as well as those who care about and love them, who need to know their risk and what they can do about it.

As Dr. Chodak points out, being empowered and learning to cope comes through knowledge and hope. Us TOO was founded on that principle 20 years ago and today thousands of volunteers continue to help support each other, learn, and together make their voices heard. Dr. Chodak is one of the well-informed, good guys in the battle against prostate cancer with his long history of contributions. His book provides a comprehensive view of this complex and often controversial disease.

My personal "Thank you" goes out to him.

Thomas N. Kirk
President and Chief Executive Officer
Us TOO International
Prostate Cancer Education and
    Support Network
Downers Grove, Illinois

Introduction

Why This Book Will Help You Win the Battle

If you or a loved one has been diagnosed with prostate cancer, many emotions and questions probably are going through your head.

- Can the cancer be treated?

- Which is the best treatment?

- How much will the treatment affect your quality of life?

- Will the treatment make it possible to watch your children and grandchildren grow up?

Winning the Battle Against Prostate Cancer will provide easy-to-understand answers to these and many other key questions.

When you and your family members begin to research this topic, confusion often occurs. There are so many opinions on what to do and too much information to read. Searching for the words "prostate cancer treatments" on the Internet will show more than 16 million hits. Advertisements for many treatments are common. This raises even more questions.

- Which of these Internet sites are useful?

- Is the information accurate and up to date?

- How can you tell which ones are biased?

- Which Internet sites can you trust?

Winning the Battle Against Prostate Cancer is a one-stop source that provides up-to-date, accurate, and balanced information about every stage of this disease. It will do away with the confusion caused by reading many of those Internet sites.

You are probably not aware that prostate cancer is a very different cancer than others such as colon or lung cancer. The following are some differences between a prostate cancer and a colon or lung cancer:

- Those cancers are always life threatening whereas prostate cancer often is not.

- Those cancers must be treated aggressively whereas many prostate cancers never need to be treated.

- Those cancers have a limited number of treatments whereas prostate cancer has many options.

- Most doctors agree on how to manage those cancers but they do not agree on how to manage prostate cancer.

Too often, doctors recommend a treatment for prostate cancer based on their personal choice rather than because of good medical studies. Also, many doctors fail to explain the pros and cons of every option available. The list of biases about this disease is quite long and it includes the following:

- Surgeons are more likely to recommend surgery whereas radiation therapists will more likely recommend radiation.

- Surgeons disagree about which method for removing the prostate is the best.

- Radiation therapists disagree on which of the seven types of radiation is the best.

- Some of the treatments promoted are so new that long-term results are not available but this limitation is rarely explained.

- Every treatment can cause complications. How often they occur depends in part on the doctor doing the treatment. Unfortunately, most doctors do not know their results so they quote those reported by the "experts," which can mislead you.

- Doctors often use poorly done medical studies to support their recommendation without explaining their weaknesses.

This book will clear up the confusion by explaining what is known and what is missing for every treatment. It will help you understand the pros and cons and risks and benefits of each treatment without any bias. If medical studies are available, they will be explained so you will understand what is good and bad about them. Just because a study is published in a medical journal does not mean the information is always good or correct. Some studies are much more reliable than others.

Another strength of this book is its firm adherence to the principles of *evidence-based medicine* or EBM. It means that a therapy will be *recommended* only when high quality scientific studies have demonstrated it *is* the best option. This book tells you which treatments have been studied in this manner. When those studies do not exist, this book will help you understand the pros and cons of all the treatments available.

This book also includes the results of many important studies published in the past 3 to 4 years. These either were not available or were overlooked when other prostate cancer books were published. These newer studies have led to many changes in how men should be treated. Although you might expect your physician to provide the latest information, few of them keep completely up to date. Hence, without this book, you may receive incorrect care and advice.

Another important feature is its ability to help you play a role in deciding what is done. You may be one of the many men who are no longer content to let the doctor decide. The challenge with prostate cancer is that the treatments can sometimes be worse than the disease. *The key is to find the treatment that is right for you.* Some men would prefer to preserve their quality of life rather than live as long as possible and others want the opposite. This is a very personal decision. How can the doctor know what matters most to you? The treatment must be tailored to meet *your needs and your goals*. To play an active role, *you need to know what you need to know*, which means asking the right questions. This book will provide the questions to ask in a way that should be acceptable to most doctors. Once you get those questions answered, you will be able to help select the treatment that is right for you.

Lastly, you may want to know what you can do on your own to improve the outcome. That may include things like changing your diet or taking herbs, vitamins, and supplements. This can be a very confusing area with many items being advised either by other patients or by promotional Web sites. Before doing anything, you should know the answers to the following questions:

- Are they helpful?

- Is there any potential harm?

- Are there good studies supporting their use or only personal stories and testimonials?

- Will they interfere with other treatments for your cancer?

This book will explain what is known and not known about all the alternative therapies being promoted so that you can make an informed decision about which one is right for you.

As you begin to read and learn about this disease, take your time and don't panic. There is no need to rush into a treatment. Your prostate cancer did not develop yesterday or last month and it does not need to be treated within the next month. Learn about all the options available and don't be afraid to ask questions. Combining that with *Winning the Battle Against Prostate Cancer* will be the best combination to achieve your goals.

Acknowledgments

This book could not have been written without the help and support of many individuals.

First and foremost is Robin Meyer, my soon-to-be wife and most special partner in life. She provided enormous emotional support and advice throughout the entire project and spent nearly as many hours critiquing the manuscript as it took for it to be written.

To my agent, Bob Silverstein of Quicksilver Books, who provided much-needed advice about creating a proposal that would move the project forward, and helped me persevere through so many disappointments.

To Terry Herbert for his countless hours critiquing this work from the perspective of an unusually well-informed patient.

To Alan Finder and Mike Scott for their helpful edits of parts of the manuscript.

To Susan B. Goodman and Beth Barry for connecting me to the right people so this project could come to life.

To Noreen Henson and Demos Health Publishing for giving me the opportunity to see this dream come true.

To the countless patients I've treated over the years, for inspiring me to find ways of improving the treatment of men with prostate cancer.

Lastly, to the many teachers who gave me the tools to distinguish the difference between good and bad science.

Winning the Battle Against Prostate Cancer

GET THE TREATMENT THAT IS RIGHT FOR YOU

I

PREVENTION, EARLY DETECTION, AND SCREENING FOR PROSTATE CANCER

Preventing Prostate Cancer

Things That May Be Good or Bad for You

Even if you already have been diagnosed with prostate cancer, this chapter still is worth reading. You may have sons, brothers, or friends who know your diagnosis and are concerned that they might get it. This chapter can provide you with useful information about preventing prostate cancer that you can give to them or perhaps still use for yourself.

Many articles in health magazines and on the Internet talk about preventing prostate cancer and other diseases using diet, herbs, vitamins, and supplements. They often refer to studies that get published in medical journals as providing "proof" they are good for you. The studies they are referring to in almost every case are called *epidemiological studies*, which unfortunately have very important weaknesses.

An epidemiological study is done by collecting information from a large number of people on such details as diet, vitamins, herbs, or supplements they take and any activities they do such as exercise or smoking. Other information collected includes their level of income and education, type of job, and details about their health. That would include diseases they have or had in the past and medications they take or have taken. This is all fed into a computer and researchers then look for anything that might be more common in people with a particular disease. Over the years, epidemiological studies reported that foods and supplements shown in the next table might lower the risk of getting prostate cancer.

Foods, Vitamins and Supplements That May Prevent Prostate Cancer

---

Omega-3 oils

Flaxseed, fish oils

Lycopene (in tomatoes and other foods)

Selenium

Vitamins A, D, and E

Green tea

Cruciferous vegetables (broccoli, cauliflower, brussel sprouts, cabbage)

Soy (genistein and daidzein)

Baked beans

Resveratrol (red wine)

Many others not on this list were found to reduce the chance of getting cancer in general, but they are not specific for prostate cancer. Epidemiological studies have also found that some things *increase* the chances of getting prostate cancer as shown in the next table.

Foods, Vitamins, and Supplements That May Increase Risk of Prostate Cancer

---

Red meat

Calcium

High glycemic index diet

High-fat diet

Often, the news media and health magazines pick up on the latest epidemiological study with a great tendency to exaggerate the results. After hearing or reading one of these stories, many individuals run out and buy whatever was highlighted in those reports. Then, sometime later another epidemiological study concludes the same thing is bad for one's health and then people don't know what to do.

Regardless of the results, these articles make it seem like an epidemiological study definitely proves that something is good or bad for you. What those articles rarely do is make you aware of their limitations or weaknesses. This leads to the following questions:

- Which epidemiological studies are you supposed to trust to give you the right information?

- What can epidemiological studies really tell us?

- What should you tell family and friends about preventing prostate cancer?

The most important message here is don't trust results from epidemiological studies because they can never prove anything. They can only suggest something is good or bad for you but they are not able to prove it is true.

The only way to prove that something truly prevents prostate cancer is to do a proper study. That requires taking a group of men and assigning them to get either the item in question or a placebo, which is something that has no affect on your body. The most important requirement of a good study is that it be randomized. It means that a computer chooses the treatment rather than the person entering or the doctor doing the study. Without this study design the results can be biased making the accuracy of the results uncertain. This study is called a prospective, randomized, controlled trial. It is the same type of study that must be done by pharmaceutical companies when they want to get a new drug on the market.

Fortunately, several prospective, randomized, controlled studies aimed at preventing prostate cancer have been done. Two of them used drugs approved by the Food and Drug Administration (FDA) for treating prostate enlargement and one study was done using over-the-counter supplements.

Preventing Prostate Cancer With Finasteride

The first study used finasteride (Proscar), a drug that affects the hormones in the prostate gland. Normally, prostate cells change the male hormone testosterone to another hormone called Dihydrotestosterone (DHT). Both of them help normal and cancerous prostate cells grow but DHT is 10 times stronger. Two proteins called type 1, 5-alpha reductase and type 2, 5-alpha reductase are needed to make DHT from testosterone. Drugs that block these proteins are called 5-alpha reductase inhibitors or 5-ARIs.

Finasteride works by blocking type 2, 5-alpha reductase. Without DHT, the prostate gland shrinks. Based on studies that showed finasteride could prevent the growth of prostate cancer in mice, doctors thought it might prevent prostate cancer in men.

The study began in 1993. Men older than age 55 could join if they had a normal prostate exam called a digital rectal exam (DRE) and a prostate-specific antigen (PSA) level below 3.0 ng/mL. PSA is an abbreviation for prostate-specific antigen, a protein produced by normal and cancerous prostate cells. The higher the PSA level, the greater the chance a man has prostate cancer.

More than 18,000 volunteers were randomized to take either a placebo or 5 mg of finasteride once a day for seven years. Once a year, everyone had a DRE and PSA test. If either one was abnormal, a prostate biopsy was done to see if that person had prostate cancer. Everyone without prostate cancer was supposed to have a prostate biopsy at the end of the study, but many refused. The study showed that finasteride prevented some men from getting diagnosed with prostate cancer. The actual results were:

- Prostate cancer was detected in 24.4% of men taking the placebo, but in only 18.4% of men taking finasteride.

- Although a greater number of fast-growing cancers were diagnosed in the group taking finasteride, doctors believe that was because of the drug shrinking the prostate, making those cancers easier to find. They do not believe finasteride makes cancers worse.

The following side effects occurred.

Side Effect	Placebo	Finasteride
Reduced volume of ejaculate	47%	60%
Decreased erections	62%	67%
Decreased sex drive	60%	65%
Breast enlargement (gynecomastia)	3%	5%
Prostate enlargement (BPH)	9%	5%
Increased urinary frequency or urgency	16%	13%
Urinary retention	6%	4%
Prostatitis	6%	4%
Urinary infection	1%	1+%

Side effects related to sexual function were more common in the finasteride group and urinary side effects were more common in the placebo group. Although the study shows finasteride does prevent prostate cancer in some men, it has been criticized because it did not answer three important questions.

- Will finasteride lower a man's chances of dying from prostate cancer? The answer to this question will take many more years of follow-up.

- How many of the cancers prevented would never have been dangerous? Because many men have a prostate cancer that would never cause any harm, preventing them will not help those men live longer or better.

- Is it necessary to continue the drug beyond seven years? Because the men in the study only took the drug for that long, it is unclear whether they must stay on the drug for the rest of their lives or the benefit will continue even if they stop the drug.

The second question is particularly important because prostate cancer is an unusual disease. It is often found when an autopsy is performed on men dying from something other than prostate cancer. In other words, it is quite common to *have* prostate cancer and much less common to *suffer* or *die* from it even when it is not treated. If the cancers prevented by finasteride would never have been dangerous, then why bother taking the drug?

Still, the study clearly proves that taking 5 mg of finasteride per day for seven years can reduce a man's chances of being diagnosed with prostate cancer. It also has other benefits. The drug can decrease the chances of having frequent urination, needing surgery to urinate and getting inflammation in the prostate.

Using this drug does have some trade-offs. For every 17 men taking it for seven years, only one avoids getting cancer. This means the other 16 are not being helped except for a small improvement in urinary function. The risks are as follows:

- About 1 out of every 13 men will have decreased fluid come out during an orgasm.

- About 1 out of 20 men will have decreased erections and decreased sex drive.

- About 1 out of 50 men will get breast enlargement.

Fortunately, most side effects go away when the drug is stopped.

So what should you say to your family and friends? The best advice is to take the drug if their goal is to do whatever possible to avoid getting prostate cancer. If they are concerned about getting a side effect, then they can try the drug for one or two months and stay on it if no side effects occur. If they get a side effect, then the drug can be stopped. The good news is, doctors finally have proof that a drug can reduce the chance of a man getting diagnosed with prostate cancer.

What Do Experts Recommend?

After the study was published, a panel of urologists from the American Urological Association (AUA) and oncologists from the American Society of Clinical Oncologists (ASCO) made the following recommendation about finasteride and another 5 ARI called dutasteride:

> Asymptomatic men with a PSA no higher than 3.0 ng/ml who are regularly screened with PSA or are anticipating undergoing annual PSA screening for early detection of prostate cancer may benefit from a discussion of the benefits of 5-ARIs for seven years for the prevention of prostate cancer and the potential risks (including the possibility of high-grade prostate cancer) to be able to make a better-informed decision.

Reducing Prostate Cancer Risk With Dutasteride

Another drug approved by the FDA for treating men with prostate enlargement is called *dutasteride* (Avodart). It also affects testosterone but blocks both type 1 and type 2, 5-alpha reductase. This study tested the drug in men who had a previous prostate biopsy that did not show cancer. This study was done for two reasons. First, doctors thought it might lower the odds of getting diagnosed with prostate cancer. Second, it also might slow down the growth of cancer in men who had cancer that was missed by the biopsy.

This also was a prospective, randomized, double-blind, controlled study. Men between the ages 55 and 70 were assigned to take a placebo or 0.5 mg of dutasteride each day for four years. Neither they nor the doctors conducting the study knew which drug was being taken. A prostate biopsy was performed two and four years after the study began. The key results were:

- Prostate cancer was diagnosed in 19.9% of the dutasteride group compared to 25% in the placebo group.

- In the third and fourth year, 12 fast-growing cancers were found in the dutasteride group compared to only one in the placebo group.

- Urinary retention occurred in 1.6% of the dutasteride group compared to 6.7% of the placebo group.

- Although heart failure was slightly more common in the treated group, the FDA does not believe it was caused by the drug.

This study shows that men with a negative biopsy who take dutasteride can reduce their risk of having a positive biopsy over the next four years. It lowered the detection rate by about 5% meaning it helped 1 out of every 20 men. Some experts are concerned that most of the cancers prevented were those usually found on autopsy and were not likely to be life threatening. Therefore, the drug was not really helping them. Another criticism is that a few more dangerous tumors were found in the dutasteride group in the third and fourth year. It could mean the drug was making some tumors worse. Lastly, doctors do no know if you must take the drug for the remainder of your life to continue to benefit or what happens if you stop the drug.

The Bottom Line About Finasteride and Dutasteride

So far, the FDA has not approved either drug for preventing or reducing the risk of prostate cancer, although they are expected to make a decision soon about dutasteride. Even so, if you want to lower your chance of getting diagnosed with prostate cancer, then taking one of these drugs is a reasonable thing to do. If you have already had a negative biopsy and are concerned about finding cancer in the future, then taking dutasteride may be worthwhile. Be aware that it is not yet know if either of them will lower your odds of dying from prostate cancer and they may cause side effects that do not always disappear after stopping the drugs.

Can Vitamin E and Selenium Prevent Prostate Cancer?

Over the years, some studies suggested that vitamin E or selenium might be able to prevent prostate cancer. To test this properly, the National Cancer Institute (NCI) sponsored a prospective, randomized study called the Selenium and Vitamin E Cancer Prevention Trial (SELECT). Men were assigned to one of the following four groups:

- vitamin E + placebo

- selenium + placebo

- vitamin E + selenium

- placebo + placebo

The study design would make it possible to see if vitamin E and selenium taken alone or together could prevent prostate cancer. The dose of selenium was 200 µg per day and the dose of vitamin E was 400 IU of *alpha-tocopherol* per day. Caucasian men older than age 55 and African American men older than age 50 were allowed to volunteer. They could enter the study only if their PSA level was less than 4.0 ng/mL.

Although the study was supposed to continue for 12 years, it was stopped after seven years because *there was no chance that either supplement given alone or both taken together would prevent prostate cancer.* That means vitamin E and selenium do not prevent prostate cancer. The study even found that men taking vitamin E might have a greater chance of getting diabetes.

The Role of Diet and Exercise in Preventing Cancer

These studies are good examples why proper testing must be done to tell if drugs or supplements are good for you. Unfortunately, most of the things listed in the "food, vitamins, and supplements" chart probably will never be tested in that way. So, what is the right message to give your family and friends about the other items on that list? Doctors estimate that about one third of all cancers are related to our diet. Many medical organizations have outlined some *dos and don'ts* regarding diet that may be good for your health as shown in the next table.

Healthy Diet Recommendations

Eat 5 cups each of fresh fruits and vegetables each day.

Avoid foods that are high in saturated fat, trans fat, and cholesterol.

Eat whole grains.

Eat lean meats, poultry without skin, fish, beans, and fat-free or low-fat milk and milk products.

Prepare foods with little salt.

Choose foods and beverages that are low in added sugar.

If you drink alcoholic beverages, do so in moderation.

Regular exercise is also important for helping to maintain your weight and promote general health. Moderate exercise is advised about five days a week. Smoking is an obvious "no-no."

Should you take vitamins and other supplements to prevent prostate cancer? Despite the number of advertisements promoting them, the best answer is *No; don't take supplements at this time* for several reasons.

- There is no proof that they really work.

- No one knows what dose would be best, what age to start, and how long to continue them.

- Many of them contain contaminants, which often are not disclosed.

- They do cause side effects of which some may be serious.

- They may reduce the effectiveness of your prescription drugs or increase the odds of having side effects from them.

Most people think that even if vitamins and supplements don't work, what's the harm? The answer to that question becomes clearer as more good studies are done. The fact is that vitamins and supplements can cause side effects and in some cases they can be dangerous. For example, vitamin E supplements were recommended for many years to promote a healthy heart and to prevent cancer. The problem is that people were seldom told that it can increase the chance of a stroke because of bleeding in the brain. Eating a healthy diet will provide the necessary amount of these agents without the need for supplements. Whether taking more than you need is good for you remains unknown.

The Bottom Line About Diet and Supplements

Men without prostate cancer who want to do something to reduce their chance of getting it can consider taking either finasteride or dutasteride. Both offer the additional advantage of reducing urinary problems. Each man must decide if the chances of benefitting are worth the cost and the chance of getting a side effect. At this time, no proof exists that anything else will prevent this disease. Taking vitamins and supplements actually could do more harm than good. Without good proof from well-done studies, they should not be used. Eating a healthy diet and having a regular exercise program are the best approaches to living a healthy life with many benefits beyond possibly preventing cancer.

Screening and Early Detection: Understanding the Risks and Benefits

What is screening? Does it save lives? Are there any risks? Should a man or his doctor decide about being screened? These are all important questions. If you already have been diagnosed with prostate cancer, do these questions really matter? The answer is *yes* because the answers may help you decide which treatment to get. It also can make it easier to talk with friends and relatives about whether they should be screened.

What Is Screening?

Screening means testing people for a disease when they don't have any symptoms. In other words, they are said to be *asymptomatic*. Screening is done to find cancers before they have spread, when they are easier to cure. Prostate cancer is more difficult to cure when a man has symptoms.

There are two ways to screen for prostate cancer, *mass screening* and *individual screening*. Mass screening means many men are invited to some location such as a hospital, church, or shopping center where a screening test is performed. Individual screening means that men are tested during a visit to their doctor. Both mass and individual screening have the same potential risks and benefits.

What Is Prostate-Specific Antigen?

You may have heard the term PSA but may not understand what it means. PSA stands for a protein called *prostate-specific antigen*, which is found in men and women. In men, it is mostly found in the prostate gland. In women, it is found in the breast and in the fluid around a fetus. Its role in women is unclear; but in men, it helps sperm fertilize a woman's egg.

PSA also is produced by prostate cancer cells located anywhere in the body. In 1986, the Food and Drug Administration (FDA) approved a blood test to monitor PSA levels of men who had been diagnosed with prostate cancer. A rise in the PSA level means the disease is getting worse and a drop means it is getting better. The level is reported as nanograms per milliliter of serum and abbreviated as ng/mL. The equivalent of one nanogram is one-billionth of a gram and 1 milliliter is equivalent to one-thousandth of a liter.

Using Prostate-Specific Antigen to Help Detect Prostate Cancer

Before the PSA test was developed, the only way a doctor could test for prostate cancer was to perform a *digital rectal exam* or DRE. This was done by wearing a rubber glove and placing the index finger into the rectum. Because the prostate gland is next to the rectum (see Chapter 4), doctors can feel the prostate gland through the rectal wall. Finding a lump, an odd shape or hardness, could mean a man has prostate cancer. The problem with the DRE is that most cancers it finds are outside the prostate, which is harder to cure.

Several years after the PSA test was approved to monitor prostate cancer, doctors began to use it with the DRE to detect prostate cancer. Both tests were done on men who urinated slowly or woke up at night to urinate. Those symptoms could be caused by prostate enlargement or prostate cancer. Doctors believed that a PSA level up to 4 ng/mL was normal. A prostate biopsy was recommended if either the DRE or the PSA was abnormal. A biopsy was needed because an elevated PSA also can occur for reasons other than prostate cancer, as shown in the following table.

Noncancerous Causes of an Abnormal PSA

---

1. Prostate enlargement (BPH or benign prostate hypertrophy)

2. Inflammation in the prostate (prostatitis)

3. Prostate infection

4. Trauma to the prostate

Using Prostate-Specific Antigen to Screen for Prostate Cancer

The success of PSA to help diagnose prostate cancer led doctors to use it as a screening test in men without symptoms. Prostate cancer was diagnosed in one out of every four men with a PSA between 4 ng/mL and 10 ng/mL even when the DRE was normal. The good news was most of them had curable tumors. In the early 1990s, many doctors and medical organizations began to advise that all men be screened with a PSA starting at age 50. Men with a high risk for this cancer were advised to begin testing at age 40 or 45.

Each year this was done, the PSA diagnosed an increasing number of men with early-stage cancer and a decreasing number with advanced cancer. Many doctors viewed this as a real benefit to men's health. Others said that finding more early-stage cancers is important, but it does not prove that screening saves lives. Without proof it truly helps, men should not be told that screening was a good thing to do. It might even be causing more harm than good.

Why Screening Is Controversial

At first, it may seem odd to hear that screening is controversial. After all, if screening finds more curable cancers, then why doesn't that prove screening is a good thing to do? According to experts, finding more curable cancers is not enough. *Screening also must increase survival and reduce the number of men dying and/or suffering from the disease.* The only way to prove screening saves lives is by doing a randomized study.

The reason this debate continued for about 20 years is that no good study had ever been completed. Then, in March 2009, results from two randomized screening studies were published. Both of them began more than 10 years ago and it took that long to get any results.

The study done in the United States enrolled men between the ages of 55 and 74 and assigned them to have a PSA and DRE every year for six years. The control group only had routine care by their personal doctors. The study confirmed that screening detects more early-stage prostate cancers compared to men not being screened. After 10 years, however, the death rate from prostate cancer was not affected. In other words, *the study did not prove that screening saves lives.*

There were some problems with the study. The main one is that not all men did what they were supposed to do. Many men who were assigned to the "control group" actually were screened, whereas some men who were assigned to be tested refused to do it. Thus, the study turned out to be screening *some* men compared to screening *most* men. Although the study is negative so far, more time is needed before any firm conclusions can be made. It still is possible that screening will lower the death rate from prostate cancer when these men are followed for a longer period of time.

The second study was performed in several European countries. It differed from the study done in the United States in several ways.

- It was much larger than the American study.

- It included men between 55 and 69 years old.

- The screened men only had a PSA test done every four years without a routine DRE.

- Each country followed a slightly different protocol.

This study found that screening did lower the death rate from prostate cancer by about 20% over the course of nine years. Many people believe that even more men will benefit with longer follow-up. *This study is the first proof that screening does save lives.* The problem is that the chance of benefitting is small and there are risks.

SUMMARY OF EUROPEAN SCREENING STUDY

To prevent one man from dying of prostate cancer, about 1,000 men had to be screened for nine years and between 24 and 48 men had to be treated. This means many men were getting a treatment that caused side effects but did not help increase their survival.

In July 2010, another report was published that included some of the men who were also part of the European study. The difference is they were followed for 14 years and the benefit from screening was greater. All men between the ages of 50 and 64 were identified in the city of Göteborg, Sweden. In this study, 10,000 of these men were contacted and offered a PSA test every two years until they reached the age of 71. Another 10,000 were identified but not contacted. They were followed to see how many eventually were diagnosed with prostate cancer and what happened to them. The study found the following:

- Prostate cancer was the cause of death in 9 out of every 1,000 men who were not screened compared to only 5 of every 1,000 men who were screened. This means screening lowered the death rate from prostate cancer by 44% but only helped 0.4% of the men getting tested.

- Advanced prostate cancer was detected in 9 out of every 1,000 men who were not screened, compared to only 3 out of every 1,000 men who were screened. This means that screening reduced the chance of having advanced disease by about 67% but only helped 0.6% of the men getting screened.

- Prostate cancer was diagnosed in one out of every 234 men who were screened.

- For each man who avoided dying from prostate cancer, 15 men had to be screened, diagnosed, and treated for prostate cancer during those 14 years. This means 14 out of 15 received a diagnosis and treatment that had not helped them.

- The overall survival was not different in the two groups. This means that being screened lowered a man's risk of dying from prostate cancer but the man still went on to die of some other cause without living any longer.

- The drop in the death rate from prostate cancer did not appear until after 10 years. That means there is little reason to screen men who are not expected to live longer than 10 years.

This study is still ongoing and may show even greater benefits with longer follow-up. An important question not yet answered is, "What was the impact of screening and treatment on their quality-of-life?" That information is vital so other men can decide if the benefit of screening is worth the risk.

This study provides reasons why men should be screened and why they should not be screened.

One additional study has been published that combined the results from six randomized screening studies involving almost 400,000 men. It found that screening did not affect the chance of dying from prostate cancer nor did it help men live longer. This study makes the overall benefit of screening more uncertain. Knowing these results will enable you to make a decision whether to be tested.

You should not assume that your doctor has read these studies. Therefore, when going for a checkup, be sure to ask your doctor if he or she plans to perform a PSA test and discuss the pros and cons before it is done.

Why Don't More Men Benefit From Screening?

You might ask, "Why didn't more men benefit from getting screened and treated?" The answer is that prostate cancer is a very unusual disease. The older men get, the more likely they will have it. Autopsy studies show that by age 50, about 30% of men have cancer cells in their prostate and by age 80, it is up to 50%. Fortunately, those cancer cells will never harm most of those men and only 3% will die from it. In fact, most men will never even know they have prostate cancer unless they are screened and a biopsy is done. However, if they are screened and cancer is found, most will be treated. That means many men will get an unnecessary treatment, which happened in the European and Göteborg study. Screening found many cancers that were not dangerous but the men still were treated.

What Is the Advice From Medical Societies About Screening?

What are medical societies now saying about screening? The American Cancer Society issued a report with the message stated as follows:

2010 AMERICAN CANCER SOCIETY GUIDELINE

Men with no symptoms who have at least a 10-year life expectancy should have an opportunity to make an informed decision with their health care provider about screening for prostate cancer. This is done after receiving information about the uncertainties, risks, and potential benefits associated with screening.

The American Urological Association (AUA), the national association of urologists, made a more aggressive recommendation.

2010 AMERICAN UROLOGICAL ASSOCIATION GUIDELINE

The AUA believes that early detection of and risk assessment for prostate cancer should be offered to asymptomatic men 40 years of age or older who have a life expectancy of at least 10 years.

According to the AUA, the decision to perform a biopsy then is based in part on how much the PSA has changed from its previous test. This is a different approach from recommending a biopsy for a PSA above a certain level. You should be aware that this guideline is not based on any study proving it will save more lives than testing at age 50. It is merely an opinion voiced by the doctors on that committee. It might cause even more unnecessary treatment.

How to Screen and Who to Screen for Prostate Cancer

If you decide that screening is the right thing to do, the best advice is to have a DRE and PSA once a year starting at age 50. If you are at high risk for prostate cancer, then have your first test at age 40 or 45. The high-risk group includes African Americans and those with a father or brother who has been diagnosed with prostate cancer.

Is there an upper age limit to screening? Many people disagree about the right answer. By now, you should realize that screening helps very few men within 10 years of being tested. That means your life expectancy should be greater than 10 years for you to have a reasonable chance of benefitting from screening. One panel of experts concluded that *men who are 75 and older* should not be screened because the harms outweigh the benefits. The reason is that 75-year-old men living in the United States have an average life expectancy of only about 10 years. Most men older than 75 who are screened and diagnosed will die of something other than prostate cancer. Screening will help very few of them to live longer. They are much more likely to get a treatment they did not need and possibly get side effects they could have avoided. That does not mean you shouldn't be tested at that age. It is a decision that should be made after you understand the risks and benefits. The bottom line is that you should understand what is good and bad about screening so you can decide what to do and be able to counsel your friends and family.

Other Approaches to Screening

There is a way to reduce the risks of screening but still get the potential benefits. No rule says that you must be treated right away if cancer is detected. You could be watched very carefully to see if the cancer shows signs of getting worse and only then decide to undergo treatment. If the cancer never grows, then it would never be treated. The term used for this is active surveillance (see Chapter 10). It has been in use since 1995. So far, active surveillance appears to be a safe option allowing more than 50% of men avoid being treated.

The Bottom Line About Screening

After more than 20 years of controversy, doctors finally have some proof that screening saves lives. The problem is it comes at a big price. Screening using the PSA test has both benefits and risks. The benefit is that it may slightly lower your chance of dying from or being harmed by prostate cancer in the next 14 years. The risk is not from the test itself, but from what happens next. It could result in treatment for a cancer that would never cause any harm.

That treatment could cause permanent side effects that affect your bladder, bowel, and sexual function. Thus, screening is a gamble and you will have to decide whether the benefit is worth the risk. The following summary may help you with this decision.

SUMMARY

You *should* be screened if your goal is to lower the chance of being harmed by prostate cancer. Most men who are screened do not benefit from it.

   You *should not* be screened if your goal is to have the best quality-of-life. Not being screened will avoid unnecessary treatment and the side effects that could occur, but the risk of dying from prostate cancer is slightly higher.

The Prostate Biopsy— When, If, and How?

3

In the early 1990s, most doctors in the United States thought that a prostate-specific antigen (PSA) level less than 4 ng/mL was normal. A few years later, some said a normal PSA level was less than 2.5 ng/mL. Then, in 2003, things changed drastically. A well-done study led to biopsies on men with a normal digital rectal examination (DRE) regardless of their PSA level. Prostate cancer was diagnosed in 16% of men with a PSA level between 0 and 1 ng/mL, and 28% of men with a PSA level between 1.1 and 2 ng/mL. This has completely changed the message all men should be given about their PSA level.

KEY POINTS

1. No PSA level is *normal*.
2. The higher the PSA level, the greater the chance a man has prostate cancer.

Many doctors are not aware of this study and still think that a PSA level up to 4 ng/mL is normal. As a result, they tell their patients that a PSA level was "okay" when it is less than 4 ng/mL rather than tell them the exact number. To avoid getting the wrong information, you should always ask your doctor for a copy of the report to make sure you get the right message. Another reason to get a copy of the report is that many companies make PSA tests and the results may vary. In most cases, the test used is included in the report. Check to see whether the same test was used in case your next PSA level is different from the last one. If they are different, another PSA test should be done in a few months before you agree to have a biopsy.

When Should a Biopsy Be Performed?

Because prostate cancer can be present at any PSA level, how is the decision made to recommend that you have a biopsy? The next table shows some of the indications doctors are now using for a prostate biopsy.

Indications for a Prostate Biopsy

1. An abnormal DRE.

2. An initial PSA level greater than 2.5 ng/mL without other reasons for it to be high.

3. A rise in the PSA level of at least 0.75 ng/mL per year. This is based on three PSA tests done during a period of at least 18 months.

4. A doubling of the PSA in three years or less.

This table is a general guide and not a strict set of rules. A biopsy usually is recommended if your doctor feels something abnormal on the DRE even when the PSA level is low or stable. Although cancer may be present at any PSA level, most doctors do not recommend a biopsy unless the PSA is greater than 2.5 ng/mL or 3 ng/mL. Perhaps, the best way to decide about a biopsy is to compare the latest result with your previous ones. Doctors get concerned when the PSA level is going up. Some studies suggest a biopsy should be done if the PSA level increases by 0.75 ng/mL per year for two years. Another reason is if the PSA level is doubling within three years. You can determine your own PSA level doubling time using a free online cal-culator (http://www.mskcc.org/applications/nomograms/Prostate/PsaDoublingTime.aspx). You should be aware that the PSA level may go up after sexual activity or riding a bike. To be safe, both should be avoided for at least 24 hours before the test. Be sure to tell the doctor if one of them did occur. That way, the doctor will repeat the PSA test before telling you a biopsy should be done. The good news is doctors now have a better understanding of how to use the PSA test to detect prostate cancer.

Preparing for a Prostate Biopsy

There is no standard preparation for a prostate biopsy. Most doctors will advise you to stop taking any blood thinners about one week in advance, but there are no studies proving that it is necessary. Warfarin (Coumadin), vitamin E, and any nonsteroidal anti-inflam-matory drugs such as aspirin, ibuprofen, or naproxen fall into that group. You can expect the doctor to give you an enema when you're in the office or tell you to take one before arriving. The reasons for doing it are to lower the chance of getting an infection and make it easier for the doctor to see your prostate with the ultrasound.

How Is a Biopsy Performed?

A short time before the biopsy starts, an antibiotic is given to fur-ther lower the chances of getting an infection. Usually, this is a pill, but an injection may also be done. It is best to get the drug about 20 to 30 minutes before starting the biopsy to allow it to get into your bloodstream.

The procedure begins by placing you on your side on an exam table. Because the biopsy can cause some pain, doctors use different methods to make you comfortable. Some will put a gel into the rec-tum that has a pain reliever in it. Others will do a nerve block. This is done by putting the ultrasound probe into your rectum and insert-ing a small needle through the skin near the rectum. The ultrasound is used to guide the needle to the area near the right and left side of your prostate and then a pain reliever is injected. Good studies have shown that the injection does a better job at preventing pain than the gel. For that reason, make sure to ask your doctor which method will be used before scheduling your biopsy. If the standard approach is to only use the gel, you might consider seeing another doctor or request that an injection be used.

The biopsy can be done in two ways. A *transrectal biopsy* means that the needle is placed through the rectum, and a *transperineal biopsy* means that the needle is inserted through the skin in front of the rectum. The transrectal approach is done most often because it causes less discomfort and the infection rate is very low. Both methods use an ultrasound probe in the rectum that helps direct the needle into the prostate. Before the needle is inserted, it may be placed into a special biopsy "gun." When fired, the needle is pushed into the prostate about 2 in. and then pulled back very quickly, making a loud popping sound. The needle removes a small cylinder or *core* of tissue. The needle is taken out of the rectum and the core is removed and placed in a specimen container.

Another difference among doctors is the number of cores taken during the biopsy. Years ago, most did 6 cores, then it went to 8 and then to 10. Although some studies have shown that more cancers are found when 12 samples are taken, many doctors still do less than that amount. The critical question is where are the needles being inserted. Another question to ask before the biopsy is set up is, "how many cores do you usually take?" If it is less than 12, then you should ask, "why not do more?" If you want the best chance of finding out if you have cancer, then more than six should be done.

What Happens After the Biopsy?

After all the cores have been taken, the ultrasound is removed, and you can get dressed and go home. You should not have much discomfort and you can resume your normal activities. Some doctors will continue the antibiotic for one to three days but no study has shown it is better than using a single dose.

You will be told to watch for a fever or chills, which could mean an infection has developed. If either occurs, make sure to alert your doctor. This usually occurs within a few days of the biopsy. Another possible side effect is the appearance of blood in the urine or semen. It could happen within a few days or even four to six weeks later. In rare cases, a substantial amount of bleeding occurs, and a blood transfusion may be needed. The biopsy should be available in 48 hours, but doctors often will tell you it takes much longer. You can request getting the result more quickly, but it may mean you will be told over the telephone.

Who Needs a Second Biopsy?

If the biopsy doesn't show cancer, could you still have prostate cancer? The answer is yes; it could have been missed. That is why you will be told to have another PSA test in about six months. If it rises, another biopsy might be suggested. Opinions vary on how much the PSA level must rise before recommending another biopsy. Cancer is found in about one of ten men having a second biopsy.

What Is the Free PSA?

Some doctors use another test to decide when a second biopsy should be done. It is called the Free PSA. That doesn't mean you can avoid paying for it. It is just a different type of PSA test. Studies have found that PSA is present in the blood stream in several forms. Some of them attach to other proteins in the blood. They are called bound or complexed PSA. The forms of PSA that do not bind to other proteins are called free PSA. Normal prostate cells mostly make free PSA and cancer cells mostly make bound PSA. The test is reported as the percentage of free PSA out of the total. Doctors use different free PSA levels to recommend another biopsy. Some do it when the free PSA level is as high as

24% and others do it only if the free PSA level is less than 18% or 12%. The test is not perfect. Some men have cancer when the free PSA is greater than 24% and many do not have cancer when it is less than 12%.

Should you have a free PSA after one negative biopsy? At first, doctors only used it when the total PSA level was between 4 and 10 ng/mL. Now, some studies have also found it useful at any PSA level. You should ask the doctor if it will be used.

Suppose you have a second biopsy and it also is negative, is a third one ever necessary? Again, the answer is yes. Some men undergo four to six biopsies for a rising PSA level before cancer is detected or the doctor says no more is needed.

What Are Saturation Biopsies?

Saturation biopsies is the term used when more than 12 biopsies are taken. Often, 20 to 30 cores are done with this approach under a general anesthesia. Some doctors do them when a second or third biopsy is needed. The benefit of saturation biopsies is that it is less likely to miss a cancer. However, there is also a higher risk it will find a cancer that would never be dangerous. This procedure is still controversial with no good studies proving it is a better thing to do, but it is an option if you want more reassurance that you do not have prostate cancer.

Does a Biopsy Always Provide a Clear Result?

In some cases, a biopsy shows neither normal cells nor prostate cancer. Instead, the result is atypical small acinar proliferation (ASAP) or high-grade prostatic intraepithelial neoplasia (HGPIN or PIN3). Some doctors consider these results to be similar but they are not. A diagnosis of ASAP means the pathologist sees abnormal cells but is not willing to definitely call it cancer. The number of these cells is so low that the pathologist cannot be sure if cancer is present. It would be far better for you to have a repeat biopsy than to have a treatment that might be unnecessary. In fact, that is the recommended approach; repeat the biopsy within three to six months because prostate cancer will be diagnosed in about 40% to 60% of these cases. An alternative is to have a specialist review the slides.

The management of HGPIN or PIN3 has changed in the past few years. Previously, when doctors took six cores of tissue, they thought these often were present in men with prostate cancer so a repeat biopsy was advised within a few months. The approach has changed in the past few years because doctors now take 12 cores. When more are taken, the chance of finding cancer on a repeat biopsy is no different than when the initial biopsy is normal. For that reason, men can be followed without the need for a repeat biopsy unless the PSA goes up by 0.75 ng/ml per year or the prostate exam becomes abnormal.

What should be done if both HGPIN and ASAP are found? The same approach should be followed as for men with asap alone. The biopsy should be repeated within three to six months.

Because not all doctors are aware of this result, you should ask for a copy of your biopsy report. That way, you can make sure you're getting the right advice.

What Happens if the Biopsy Shows Cancer?

If the biopsy does show cancer, your doctor will decide if other tests are needed to determine which is the best treatment for you.

II

WHAT YOU NEED BEFORE GETTING TREATED

The Male Anatomy: How It All Fits Together

Before learning about your treatment options, you may benefit from an increased awareness of your anatomy and the role of each organ in your general health.

The Prostate Gland

The prostate sits in your lower pelvis, tucked behind your pubic bone, just beneath your bladder. It surrounds the *urethra*, which is the tube that carries urine from your bladder out through the tip of the penis. Directly behind the prostate is the rectum. Very little tissue separates these two organs, which is why the rectum can be injured when the prostate is being treated. Located between the prostate and rectum are the two *pelvic nerves*, which are responsible for the ability to have an erection. They also can be easily damaged during any treatment directed at the prostate. At the top of the prostate, just behind the bladder, are the two seminal vesicles.

The normal adult prostate is approximately the size of a walnut and weighs about 20 g. It has five regions or *lobes*. Prostate cancer most commonly grows in the *posterior lobe*, which is closest to the rectum. This makes it possible for your doctor to examine the prostate by placing a gloved finger inside the rectum and pushing toward the front of your body. Surrounding the prostate is a very thin layer of tissue called the *capsule*. It serves as a barrier separating the prostate from the surrounding organs. Prostate cancer may grow into or through the capsule.

The prostate gland usually increases in size as men get older, which can cause the following urinary symptoms:

- slowing of the stream,

- difficulty starting and stopping urination,

- needing to urinate during the night,

- frequent urination,

- an inability to empty the bladder, and

- dribbling.

The Urinary Bladder

Urine is made in your kidneys and passes down to your bladder through a tube called the ureter. Most people are born with two kidneys, one on the right and the other on the left, so there also are two ureters. As your bladder fills with urine, it enlarges and eventually you will begin to feel some discomfort in your lower abdomen. This is a signal that your bladder is getting full, and it is time to urinate. The average male bladder normally can hold about 300 to 400 mL before the discomfort gets severe. That is about 10 to 13 oz. The maximum capacity is about 400 to 600 mL unless the bladder has been damaged.

The reason urine stays in the bladder is because of the two muscles called the external and internal urinary sphincter. The internal sphincter is located at the bottom of the bladder. The external sphincter is located beneath the prostate and it surrounds the urethra. The external urinary sphincter is a striated muscle, like the muscles in your arms and legs. Striated muscles are under your voluntary control, which means you have the ability to tighten or relax them. The external sphincter can be strengthened by exercises, which can help decrease urinary leakage following some of the treatments for prostate cancer. The internal urinary sphincter is a *smooth* muscle like your heart. Smooth muscles work on their own, meaning you cannot control them.

The external urinary sphincter is normally contracted, which prevents urine from leaking out of your body. As your bladder fills, it sends a signal to your brain that causes the internal sphincter to relax. In response, you voluntarily tighten your external sphincter so that urine does not leak out until you decide you want to urinate. At that time, you relax your external sphincter and your bladder contracts, which forces the urine to exit from your body. These muscles may be injured by the treatments for prostate cancer.

The Seminal Vesicles

These are two small glands measuring about 5 cm in length that are located near the top of the prostate behind the bladder. The seminal vesicles play a vital role in fertility by making fluid that helps to nourish sperm cells. When you have an orgasm, the fluid from each seminal vesicle is delivered down a tube called the *ejaculatory duct* and then it passes into the urethra and out the tip of the penis.

The seminal vesicles are not needed for any other bodily function besides fertility. They are removed along with the prostate during a radical prostatectomy. The only consequence is that you will have a *dry orgasm*, which means that no fluid will come out the tip of the penis.

The Testicles

These are two egg-shaped glands located in the scrotal sac beneath the penis. The testicles have two major functions. They are responsible for making sperm cells that will fertilize a woman's egg and they produce a hormone called *testosterone*. Hormones are chemicals produced in certain organs that affect other parts of your body. Testosterone is responsible for your male characteristics such as hair growth, muscle development, your sex drive, and the growth of the prostate gland. Because this hormone also helps prostate cancer cells grow, one of the treatments is to remove the testicles, which is called *surgical castration*.

When you have an orgasm, the sperm from each testicle is released into long, thin, muscular tubes called the *vas deferens*. The end of each vas deferens joins with a seminal vesicle to form the *ejaculatory duct*. The two ducts pass through the prostate gland and join with the urethra. Following an orgasm, the sperm and seminal fluid are forced down the two ejaculatory ducts and then out through the tip of the penis. Men who no longer want to have children can have a *vasectomy* during which each vas deferens is divided. Both vas deferens also are cut when the entire prostate is removed, which makes you unable to father a child during sexual intercourse.

The Penis

This organ is responsible for sexual intercourse, and although it needs little explanation, several facts may not be known. It is made up of three columns of tissue. The two located on the sides of the penis are called the *corpus cavernosum* and the third one, called the *corpus spongiosum*, is located in between them. The tip of the penis is called the *glans* and the remainder is called the *shaft*. The corpus cavernosum and spongiosum are filled with blood vessels. When you become sexually aroused, signals are sent to the penis from the *pelvic nerves*, which cause more blood to flow into and less blood to leave the penis. This causes an erection. Following an orgasm, the blood is drained out through veins in the penis and the erection goes away.

The treatments for prostate cancer can affect the nerves and the blood vessels resulting in a decreased ability to get an erection. One of the major advances in treating men who have decreased erections has been the development of drugs that increase the blood flow into the penis, which may help improve erections.

Lymph Nodes

Lymph nodes are small glands scattered throughout the body that help fight infection. Prostate cancer can spread into the lymph nodes near the prostate by entering lymphatic channels located in the gland or they can spread to lymph nodes in other parts of the body by first entering blood vessels.

Now that you understand the basics about your anatomy, you should find it easier to understand what happens during the different treatments for your prostate cancer.

Staging Your Prostate Cancer

The best treatment for you depends on where the tumor is located. This is determined from the digital rectal examination (DRE) and from the *staging* tests described later. Before discussing the treatment options, your doctor must decide if the cancer is completely contained within the prostate, growing outside the prostate into the surrounding tissues or if it has spread to other parts of your body. If all the cells are inside the prostate, the tumor is *confined* or *localized*. Tumors growing into the surrounding tissues are called *locally advanced* and if it has spread elsewhere it is called *metastatic*. None of the staging tests is 100% accurate. They all have *false-positive* and *false-negative* results. A result is called false-positive if it appears to show the cancer has spread when it really has not. A false-negative means the test fails to recognize that the cancer really has spread.

The Bone Scan

A bone scan is the best test to find out if cancer has spread to the bones although it, too, is not 100% accurate. The false-positive and false-negative rates are about 3%. A *negative scan* means there is no evidence of cancer in the bones and a *positive scan* means something is seen on the scan that should not be there. It could be from cancer, but other things also can make it positive such as an injury.

Either a simple x-ray, a computed axial tomography (CAT) scan, magnetic resonance imaging (MRI), or a bone biopsy will be done to find out what is causing the abnormality.

A bone scan is performed by first injecting a small amount of a radioactive drug into a vein. It passes through the bloodstream and into the bones. The drug will remain in an abnormal bone and can be viewed on the scan as a *hot spot*.

The actual scan is done with you lying on a table for 1–2 hours while a special camera takes pictures. The test causes no pain except for the discomfort of lying on a hard table. Less than 1% of men get an allergic reaction to the injected material. When the test is done, you can immediately resume your normal activities.

Who Should Have a Bone Scan?

The use of the bone scan as a staging test for prostate cancer has changed over the last 10 years because of the prostate-specific antigen (PSA) test. If the value is less than 20 ng/mL, only 3 out of 1,000 men will have bone metastases but 39 will have an abnormal scan. That means you are much more likely to have an abnormal scan caused by something other than prostate cancer. The problem is you will need additional tests to find out what caused the abnormal test. Most doctors no longer order the test unless the PSA is at least 10 ng/mL or the biopsy shows an aggressive cancer but the best approach probably is to do it only if the PSA is above 20 ng/mL.

Some doctors still think a bone scan should be done at any PSA level because they do not want to miss even a single case of cancer in the bones. Others do it just to get a baseline in case a bone scan is needed in the future. The problem is that too many men will be getting a test they did not need. If your doctor wants to order a bone scan, you should discuss it first so you can avoid an unnecessary test. A bone scan is worth doing if you are having any pain in your bones.

Computed Axial Tomography

A test that has greatly helped doctors care for patients is the *computed axial tomography, or CAT scan*. It takes a series of x-rays spaced small distances apart and uses a computer to create a 3-dimensional picture. A CAT scan is done to look for cancer in the lymph nodes, but it also may tell if cancer has spread into the area around the prostate. The test often is unable to detect small amounts of cancer, meaning it gives many false-negative results.

The CAT scan requires that the bowels must be cleansed. You will have to drink about 4 quarts of a liquid that will cause frequent bowel movements. It is taken until only clear fluid appears in the toilet. Before the test begins, special dye is put into the rectum and some is injected into a vein in the arm. You then lie on a table while the pictures are taken, which takes about one hour to complete.

Who Should Have a CAT Scan?

The CAT scan also was done in most men with prostate cancer before the PSA became available. Now, most doctors do not order the test when the PSA is less than 20 ng/mL. At that level, the odds of a CAT scan finding cancer in the lymph nodes are less than 1%. If the PSA is above that level, some doctors will order the scan but even then it is not very accurate. If you decide to have radiation, either a CAT scan or an MRI will be needed to plan where to deliver the treatments. If you decide to have a different treatment and have a low PSA, a CAT scan makes little sense and should not be done.

Magnetic Resonance Imaging (MRI)

Another test used by some physicians is the MRI test. Like the CAT scan, the goal of this test is to see if cancer has spread outside your prostate or into the surrounding lymph nodes. The MRI uses a strong magnetic field to give detailed images of your body. It differs from a CAT scan in two ways. The MRI does not use x-rays and no preparation is needed before the test is done. Normally you lie on a table that moves into a tunnel and then the pictures are taken. The MRI is done in less than one hour.

Some doctors now are ordering an *endorectal MRI*. It is done by placing a special probe into the rectum. At present, there is not enough proof that the endorectal MRI should be done routinely but research is ongoing to find out.

Who Should Have an MRI?

The answer is most men do not need it for two reasons. The first is the same reason for not doing a CAT scan. The chance of having cancer in the lymph nodes is very low when the PSA is under 20 ng/mL. The second reason is the test that will give many false-positive or false-negative results. The bottom line is the MRI will not really help determine which is the best treatment for you. For that reason, you should not have it until the accuracy improves.

The Prostascint Scan

This test uses antibodies and a small amount of radioactive material that attach to a protein on the surface of prostate cancer cells. It has the ability to find prostate cancer cells anywhere in the body. The problem is it too has many false-positive and false-negative results.

No food should be eaten for eight hours before the test. Prior to the scan, an enema is used to clean the bowel. The test is done by first injecting the radioactive material into a vein. Then you are placed on a table and pictures are taken with a special camera. The scan takes about one to two hours but you must return three or four days later to have another scan done. There is a very small risk of an allergic reaction to the injection.

Who Should Have a Prostascint Scan?

Although its accuracy has improved, not many doctors use this test for men with newly diagnosed prostate cancer because it gives too many false-positive and false-negative results. It may be more useful when the PSA is rising after a radical prostatectomy but at this time, few men will benefit from having this test.

What is a Ploidy Analysis?

When doctors look under the microscope at a biopsy, they cannot be sure if the cancer will grow slowly or fast. A test that may be useful is called a *ploidy analysis*. It measures the amount of genetic material, called DNA that is contained in the cells. *Diploid* cells have a normal amount of DNA and *aneuploid* cells have more DNA than normal. Weak studies suggest that aneuploid tumors are more likely to recur after treatment than diploid tumors. For that reason, some doctors recommend a more aggressive treatment if an aneuploid tumor is found but this is not supported by good studies.

The test does not require the patient to do anything. It can be done on the biopsy specimen used to diagnose the cancer. The sample is stained with certain chemicals and then put through a machine that measures the amount of DNA in the cells.

Who Should Have a Ploidy Analysis?

This study was more popular several years ago but now is rarely used. The problem with the test is that no study has shown a benefit from treating aneuploid tumors differently than treating diploid tumors. The result of this test does not help decide which treatment is best. The bottom line is this test is not worth doing.

Summary of Staging Tests

A summary of the various staging tests is provided here.

Test	Information Provided By Test	Who Should Have Test
Bone scan	Determines if prostate cancer has spread to the bones	1. Presence of bone pain 2. PSA greater than 20 ng/mL
CAT scan	Determines if cancer has spread to the seminal vesicles, lymph nodes, or other abdominal organs	1. Needed before radiation therapy 2. PSA greater than 20 ng/mL
MRI	Determines if cancer is growing outside the capsule or into seminal vesicles	Test not needed but can be done instead of CAT scan if radiation is planned
Endorectal MRI		Not needed unless accuracy improves
Prostascint scan	Determines if cancer is in lymph nodes	Test not needed
Ploidy analysis	Predict odds tumor will spread	Test not needed

Understanding Tumor Stage and Tumor Grade

The Stages of Prostate Cancer

Each man with prostate cancer is assigned a *tumor stage* and a *tumor grade*. The tumor stage is where the cancer is located in your body. Doctors can assign you a *clinical tumor stage* and a *pathologic tumor stage*. The clinical tumor stage is where doctors think your cancer is located. It is determined from the digital rectal examination (DRE), the biopsy, and any staging tests that were done. Doctors use these tools to estimate the *pathological tumor stage*, which is the true location of your cancer. The only way to know the pathological stage is by doing an autopsy. Doctors will tell you the best options for treating your cancer based on where they think your cancer is located.

Different methods are used to define the tumor stage. The *TNM Classification of Malignant Tumors* (TNM) and *Whitmore-Jewett system* are used most often in the United States. In the TNM system, T (tumor) represents the extent of cancer in the prostate gland, N (node) is for the lymph nodes, and M (metastasis) is for its presence in other parts of the body.

The following table shows a description of all the tumor stages for both staging systems.

Clinical T Stage	Whitmore–Jewett Equivalent Stage	Description
T1	A	Cancer is located inside the prostate. The DRE is normal.
T1a	A1	Cancer is found in less than 5% of the tissues removed during an operation to improve urination. The DRE is normal.
T1b	A2	Cancer is found in more than 5% of the tissues removed during an operation to improve urination. The DRE is normal.
T1c	B0	Cancer is found on a biopsy done because of an abnormal PSA test. The DRE is normal.
T2	B	DRE shows cancer inside the prostate.
T2a	B1	DRE shows cancer in less than 50% of one side of the prostate.
T2b	B1	DRE shows cancer in more than 50% of one side of the prostate.
T2c	B2	DRE shows cancer on both sides of the prostate.
T3	C	DRE shows cancer outside the prostate.
T3a	C1	DRE shows cancer outside the prostate on either right or left side.
T3b	C2	DRE shows cancer outside the prostate on both right and left sides.
T3c	C3	DRE shows cancer into one or both seminal vesicles.

Clinical T Stage	Whitmore-Jewett Equivalent Stage	Description
T4a	C	DRE shows cancer in the bladder, the rectum, or the muscle that prevents urine from leaking.
T4b	C	DRE shows cancer in the pelvic wall or pelvic muscles.

DRE indicates digital rectal examination; PSA, prostate-specific antigen.

The N stages for the lymph nodes are shown in the next table. The only way to determine if cancer is definitely in the lymph nodes is to remove them. Neither a biopsy of the lymph nodes nor a computerized axial tomography (CAT) or magnetic resonance imaging (MRI) scan is 100% accurate.

N Stage	Whitmore-Jewett Equivalent Stage	Description
Nx	D0	The status of the lymph nodes is not known, stage D0 means the PSA level is rising, but no metastases are found.
N0		Cancer is not in the lymph nodes.
N1	D1	Cancer is present in one lymph node less than 2 cm in diameter.
N2	D1	1. Cancer is in one lymph node between 2 and 5 cm in diameter. 2. Cancer is in more than one lymph node less than 5 cm in diameter.
N3	D1	Cancer in lymph nodes is greater than 5 cm in diameter.

The following table shows the M stages that represent tumor in other parts of the body. This is determined from the bone scan, CAT scan, MRI scan, x-rays, or biopsies.

M Stage	Whitmore-Jewett Equivalent Stage	Description
Mx		The status of metastases is unknown.
M0		No evidence of metastases.
M1	D2	Cancer has metastasized to other organs.
M1a		Cancer has spread into lymph nodes above the division of the aorta.
M1b		Cancer has spread into the bones.
M1c		Cancer has spread into other organs either with or without spread into the bones.

Doctors put the stages into different groups. *Localized disease* includes stages T1, N0, M0 or T2, N0, M0 in the TNM system or stages A and B in the Whitmore-Jewett system. *Locally advanced disease* is for stages T3, N0, M0 and T4, N0, M0, or stage C, and *Metastatic disease* includes N1, N2, N3 or M1 disease, or stage D.

Tumor Grade

The tumor grade describes the appearance of the cancer cells when viewed under a microscope. Like tumor stage, more than one system is used. The *Gleason Scoring System*, named for Dr. Donald Gleason, is used most often in the United States. After looking at many biopsies, he saw five types of prostate cancer cells. He scored them Gleason grade 1 if they looked almost like normal prostate cells and Gleason grade 5 if they looked nothing like normal cells. Grades 2,

3, and 4 looked increasingly abnormal. Because many biopsies showed more than one type, each patient was given two numbers. The first one is the grade of the most common cell type and the second number is the grade of the second most common cell type. When a biopsy has only one cell type, the Gleason grade is doubled. The two numbers then are added together to give the Gleason score.

Using this system, the lowest Gleason score is $1 + 1 = 2$, and the highest score is $5 + 5 = 10$. A Gleason score of 6 is the most common one for new cases of prostate cancer. The higher the Gleason score, the more dangerous is the cancer and the greater is the chance the cancer has spread or eventually will spread outside the prostate. This grading system has both strengths and weaknesses. The strengths are the following:

- It can be used to predict the response to some treatments.

- It can be used to tell if the cancer has spread outside the prostate.

Its weaknesses are the following:

- The Gleason score on the biopsy can be different from the score given after the prostate has been removed. This happens in about 20% to 30% of the cases.

- The Gleason score can vary depending on the doctor who reads it. Two pathologists reading the same biopsy will give different Gleason scores in about 20% to 30% of the cases. Even the same pathologist will give a different score 20% of the time, if asked to read the biopsy a second time.

To get the most reliable results, many doctors will send the biopsy to a lab that specializes in reading prostate biopsies. Two noted places are Bostwick Laboratories (www.bostwicklaboratories.com/home/) and Dr. Jonathan Epstein at Johns Hopkins Hospital (jepstein@jhmi .edu). You or your doctor can request a second opinion by contacting those labs.

Clinical Versus Pathological Stage

As stated earlier, the clinical stage is not always the same as the pathological stage. If doctors knew for sure where your cancer was located, you could get better advice on how to be treated. Fortunately, there is a way to get a good idea about the pathological stage of your cancer.

Doctors at Johns Hopkins Hospital created the *Partin tables* that predict the true T, N, and M stage. Although some doctors will use these tables, many do not. It is worth looking at them to help you get the right treatment. If your doctor does not give you this information, you can find it out yourself because the Partin tables are available on the Internet at no charge (http://urology.jhu.edu/prostate/partintables.php). The information you will need to determine your pathological stage can be obtained by asking the doctor for your Gleason score, T stage, and PSA level. These tables will tell you the chance that your cancer is outside the prostate, into the seminal vesicles, and into the lymph nodes.

One example is shown as follows for a man with a PSA level between 4.1 and 6 ng/mL, a clinical stage of T1c, and a Gleason score of 6.

True Location of Cancer	Percentage of Patients With This Result
All cancer is inside prostate gland	81%–85%
Some cancer is growing outside the prostate	14%–17%
Cancer is growing into seminal vesicles	1%
Cancer has spread to the lymph nodes	0%

This patient has a very high chance that his prostate cancer is contained in the prostate capsule and a very low chance that cancer is in his seminal vesicles or lymph nodes. After you know the grade and stage of your cancer, you can begin to learn about the treatment options that are best.

Understanding Medical Studies so You Can Get the Treatment That Is Right for You

Introduction

As you learn about the options for treating your prostate cancer, you may turn to reviewing medical studies. They will tell you the proportion of men who are alive, have a stable prostate-specific antigen (PSA), or did not develop widespread cancer several years after being treated. Because they are all published in medical journals, you probably will assume that they must be well done and the results must be reliable. Unfortunately, that is far from the truth. *The fact is, a great many of the studies that get published are not well done.* That means the results are unreliable. Without understanding what makes a study good or bad and how results are reported, you run the risk of not getting the treatment that is right for you.

Medical studies are done in different ways. The most common types used for prostate cancer are the following:

- A prospective, randomized, controlled study

- A prospective cohort study

- A case control, retrospective study

- An epidemiological study

What Is a Prospective, Randomized, Controlled Study?

This type of study is by far the best because it gives the most reliable information. To understand the reason, you must first know what each word means.

- *Prospective* means the study was carefully designed before anyone was treated.

- *Randomized* means that at least two treatments are being compared to each other and neither the patient nor the doctor can choose what treatment to receive. A computer will make this decision. Randomly assigning people to their treatment reduces the chance that the results will be biased or incorrect.

- *Controlled* means only patients with specific characteristics are allowed to enter the study and everyone is supposed to be managed in the same way. They all get the same tests before and after they are treated and the treatments are standardized. For example, if surgery is being compared to external radiation, every patient in the radiation group gets the same amount of radiation and it is delivered using the same technique.

When done properly, a *prospective, randomized, controlled study is the only reliable way to prove that one treatment is as good, better, or worse than another treatment*. All new drugs must be tested in this way to gain approval from the Food and Drug Administration (FDA). Unfortunately, prospective, randomized, controlled studies are very expensive to do and they can take many years to complete. That partly explains why such studies rarely have been done to compare the different treatments for prostate cancer. Without these studies, doctors are unable to determine which therapy is best.

What Is a Cohort Study?

A cohort study also is prospective, but it differs from a random-ized study in that all the individuals get to choose their treatment. For example, if a doctor wants to study the effect of a radical pros-tatectomy, any man healthy enough to undergo an operation can decide to participate. Specific information about each person is recorded and then they are followed to see what happens to them. The results are compared with other treatments published in medical journals.

Cohort studies are easier to do than prospective, randomized, controlled studies, which is partly the reason why more of these studies are done. The problem with comparing cohort studies is that the results can be very biased leading to incorrect conclusions. Using these results to compare different treatments may *suggest* that they are similar, but only a prospective, randomized study can prove if that is true.

What Is a Retrospective, Case Control Study?

This study design collects information from medical records about men who had their treatment sometime in the past. The results are then analyzed and compared to other studies. The value of retro-spective studies is that they are relatively easy to do, are not very costly, and can give immediate information without having to wait many years to get results. Unfortunately, retrospective studies often lead to incorrect conclusions for several reasons:

- There is no way to be sure that the information entered into the chart is correct. Errors are common and there is no way to correct them.

- Because the study was not prospective, patients may not have been treated in exactly the same way. For example, in a ret-rospective study of men having a radical prostatectomy, some of them also may have received radiation or hormone therapy. Combining them with men only having surgery will distort the results.

- Some men having the treatment may be excluded because of missing information. This creates a selection bias, which can make the results appear better than if all the treated patients were included.

- Allowing men to select their treatment also can create a bias, making the results appear better than if a randomized study was done.

- When the results of two retrospective studies are compared, the characteristics of the patients rarely are the same, which can lead to misleading conclusions. It would be like trying to compare apples to oranges to decide which fruit is sweeter.

As a result of these potential weaknesses, *the results of case control, retrospective studies cannot be used to make reliable conclusions.* This does not mean that the results are definitely wrong, but there is no way to be sure that they are correct. For that reason, you should use caution when told about the results of a retrospective study.

What Is an Epidemiological Study?

This also is a retrospective look at what happened to a group of individuals treated in the past. Information is collected from the medical records and then fed into a computer. It searches for anything that separates individuals into those who did well and those who did poorly. For example, consider a group of men who were all treated in the past by external radiation. When the results are analyzed, the study may find a higher survival rate in men who took vitamin C compared to those not taking it. The study would then conclude that vitamin C improves survival of men having external radiation.

Is this conclusion valid? Does it mean that men having radiation should be advised to take vitamin C to improve their survival? The answer is *no*, it is not a valid conclusion or recommendation. Epidemiological studies can *suggest* vitamin C *may* be beneficial but only a prospective, randomized, controlled trial can prove if that is true. There can be many other explanations why some men did better than others that have nothing to do with taking this vitamin.

Epidemiological studies are much easier to do than prospective, randomized, controlled studies, and they are often mentioned in the news. The problem is that the results are made to appear reliable and the weakness of the study design is rarely reported. The bottom line is you should be very cautious when making decisions based on epidemiological studies.

The Bottom Line About Medical Studies

The main message here is that some results reported to you come from well-designed studies and other results come from poorly designed studies. The better the study design, the more you can trust the results. As you learn about the different treatments in this book, you will be told what kind of study was done to arrive at the result. You will be made aware of any weaknesses that could bias the results. This is intended to help you decide which treatment is right for you.

III

HOW TO TREAT CLINICALLY LOCALIZED PROSTATE CANCER

Overview of Treatment Options

8

As you begin reading about the options for treating your prostate cancer, please be patient. The good news is that you have many options. The challenge you face is that a good study has only compared two of them, which will make your choice more difficult. The best approach is to take your time learning what is good and bad about every option. Fortunately, there is no urgency to be treated right away. Your cancer probably has been in your body for several years. It is not likely to get worse in a few weeks or even a few months while you learn about each option. You can begin this process by thinking about these questions as you do your homework.

- Which options are appropriate for your age, health, tumor stage, Gleason score, and prostate-specific antigen (PSA)?

- What is the chance each treatment will cure you?

- What are the chances your cancer will recur?

- What are the chances you will need additional treatment?

- What are all the complications or side effects that can occur?

- What are the odds you will get these complications?

Without getting the answers, you will find it hard to make a truly informed choice. It would be like playing a game called "blind poker." The rules are quite simple. The dealer gives you five cards and takes five for himself. Now you must decide how much money to bet. The problem is, you are not allowed to see any of your cards. You must play the game as if you're blind. How much would you be willing to bet without a clue about your odds of winning and losing? Clearly, if you knew you were holding four aces, you might think the odds of winning are very high. In that case, you would be willing to place a very large bet. On the contrary, you probably would save your money and fold if you had a very poor hand.

Deciding on a treatment for prostate cancer sometimes may feel like you are playing a game with similar rules. You are told about the options and maybe the possible side effects are listed but you are not given the odds of "winning" and "losing." Instead of betting money, you are betting with your survival and quality-of-life. Unless you are comfortable playing "blind," choosing the right treatment requires finding out the odds of surviving and getting side effects. Then you can decide if the benefits are worth the risks.

More than ever, treatment for prostate must be individualized. The right choice for some men may not be the right choice for you. Your goals and fears are likely to be different than those of other men. One thing to remember is every treatment offers a "package deal" of good and bad results. To get the potential benefits of a treatment, you have to be willing to accept the chance of getting side effects. The specific side effects and how often they occur may be more acceptable to you with some treatments but not others.

Too often, doctors will tell you what side effects can occur but not the percentage of men who get them. To make an informed decision and avoid playing "blind poker," you need answers to the following questions.

Information Needed About Side Effects

---

1. How often does each complication occur in men of similar age and health as your own?

2. Are the complication rates specific to your doctor or are they from some expert?

3. Was the information obtained from validated surveys, or did the doctor "estimate" the results?

4. How long does each complication last?

5. If a complication does occur, how is it treated and how often does it go away?

6. How is your quality-of-life affected by each complication?

Don't be surprised to find out that your doctor does not have this information. Most of them do not keep track of their own results so they give you an estimate or tell you what the experts report. One factor that definitely affects the results is the experience of the physician. Studies show that doctors who treated a small number of men had a higher rate of complications than doctors with more experience. Although written surveys are the most accurate way to obtain results, few doctors use them. Instead, they make an estimate, which is very inaccurate. Don't be afraid to ask your doctor these questions, otherwise you will be playing "blind poker."

Suppose you ask for a doctor's results and are told they only can be estimated. Should you get a different doctor? Not necessarily, but it certainly should be considered if you hope to do everything possible to get the best result. Without accurate answers, you have more uncertainty about what to expect from being treated by that doctor. This may make it difficult to decide if the potential benefit of a treatment is worth the potential risk of getting a complication.

The other important part of each treatment is the long-term survival results. Because prostate cancer usually grows slowly, knowing the odds of being alive at 5 or even 10 years after a treatment is not enough. Many men will live 10 years or longer even if they don't get treated. If you want to know whether a treatment is truly effective, you need results beyond 10 years. Unfortunately, the long-term results for many treatments are not known because they haven't been used long enough. Even 10-year results are not available. Without longer follow-up, there is more uncertainty about will happen to you in the future. Nothing is wrong with choosing a treatment that has only short follow-up, but you should understand that it is more of a gamble, like playing "blind poker."

In place of long-term survival, doctors use other results to compare different treatments as shown in the following table.

Potential Treatment Results

---

1. Biochemical disease-free survival—The percentage of men with a stable PSA

2. Treatment-free survival—The percentage of men not getting additional treatment

3. Metastases-free survival—The percentage of men who do not develop metastatic disease

---

Unfortunately, *none of these is a reliable substitute* for survival. These outcomes could be similar at 5 or 10 years but the survival rates at 10 or 15 years could differ. Therefore, you should be careful when reading promotions or hearing experts recommend the newer treatments based on these other results. *The truth is no one knows if any of these are an accurate predictor of long-term survival.*

If long-term survival results are not available, does it mean you should avoid that option? Not necessarily. There is nothing wrong with your choosing any treatment providing you understand that long-term results could turn out to be worse than expected. Perhaps you find something appealing about a newer treatment and you are willing to accept the uncertainty of not knowing the long-term results. The most important message is you should be as informed as possible when making your choice.

One helpful approach for comparing treatments is to divide prostate cancers into three risk groups based on their chances for causing harm. The tumor characteristics used to do this are the PSA, the Gleason score, and the clinical stage. The definitions are the following:

- Low-risk disease—Patients have a PSA less than 10 ng/mL, a Gleason score less than 7 and a clinical stage of T1 or T2a.

- Intermediate-risk disease—Patients have a PSA between 10 and 20 ng/mL, or a Gleason score of 7 or a clinical stage of T2b.

- High-risk disease—Patients have a PSA above 20 ng/mL, or a Gleason score above 7 or a clinical stage of T2c.

Low-risk tumors have a low chance of spreading in the next 10 to 15 years, and high-risk tumors have a much higher chance of spreading. Knowing which group you are in may affect which treatment is best for you.

Understanding How Medical Studies Report Results

As you begin to compare the results for different treatments, you need to be aware of the way studies report their results. In some cases, the information used by doctors may be misleading. This is best explained with some examples.

Suppose you want to know your odds of being alive 10 years after undergoing radioactive seed implantation. The doctor tells you about a study in which 100 men all received this treatment in 1999 and 80 of them were alive in 2009. That means 80% survived 10 years (80/100). This information would give you an excellent idea of what to expect from this treatment, assuming you have a similar type of tumor. Ideally, all studies would have this information but that is seldom the case.

Most studies do something different because men are treated over a number of years rather than all in the same year. That means they will have been followed for different periods. For example, suppose that out of 100 men who had a radical prostatectomy:

- 10 were treated 10 years ago.

- 20 were treated seven years ago.

- 50 were treated four years ago.

- 20 were treated only two years ago.

When doctors decide to report their 10-year results on all these men, they cannot give an *exact* result because only 10 men were followed the full 10 years. However, they can use statistical methods to *estimate* the 10-year survival rate for the entire group. In this case, the estimated 10-year survival is approximately 80%. These statistical methods will also calculate a range for the *true* result, which in this case may be 60% to 90%. This means that the true result is highly likely to be *somewhere* in that range. It could be as low as 60%, as high as 90%, or anywhere in between. Until all the men have been followed the full 10 years, the results cannot be more precise. This is very important to understand, but your doctor is very unlikely to explain it to you when you are told these results. If you ask, "What are my odds of being alive in 10 years?" You will be told "about 80%." The problem is that answer is misleading. *You should be told that, "We think the 10-year survival is 80% but it could be as low as 60% or as high as 90%.*

Now, suppose you want to know how these two treatments compare. Which one gives you the best chance of being alive in the next 10 years, surgery or seed implantation? The correct answer is, "They *appear* to give similar results *but* surgery might be better or it might be worse than the seed implantation." *There is no way to say for sure how the two treatments compare without a prospective, randomized study.*

This is the reason why comparing results from different treatments is so difficult. Almost every study published only contains *estimated* results and many have very wide ranges. That means valid comparisons can't be done and yet that is exactly what doctors try to do. You should be wary when a doctor uses estimated results to tell you that a new treatment is as good as the one that has been used much longer.

Some studies that estimate results are more helpful than are others. One that includes a large number of men followed for many years will have a narrow range for the results. Although you do not have an *exact* result, you get a pretty good idea of what to expect from that treatment. In contrast, those with a small number followed for a short time will have a very wide range. These are much more unreliable. Perhaps you may be wondering why medical journals bother publishing these weaker studies. The reason is they have to fill their pages, and good articles are in shorter supply than weaker ones. Keep this in mind as you learn about the results of different studies.

What Is "Evidence-Based Medicine"?

A growing practice around the United States is the use of evidence-based medicine. A simple definition of evidence-based medicine is "assessing the quality of medical studies that are used to counsel people about the best treatment for their disease." With this approach, a treatment can be *recommended* when prospective, randomized, controlled studies show it is better than the other options. What happens if randomized studies are not available? In that case, no treatment should be recommended as providing better results. Instead, you should be told about all the available treatments including their possible risks and benefits. Doctors still can use results from other types of studies to recommend a therapy. However, when they do this, you should be informed that it is only their personal opinion, and well-done studies have not proved it is best. This awareness will help you decide which treatment is right for you.

With this information as a foundation, the pros and cons of each treatment will now be provided. This book is not intended to promote any particular treatment unless good studies prove it is best. Rather, the goal is to enable you to make an informed choice.

Watchful Waiting

The term *watchful waiting* describes a treatment in which no therapy is given to your prostate gland and no attempt is made to cure the cancer. Instead, you are treated only if the cancer causes symptoms or if it spreads to other parts of your body. There are two reasons this therapy may be right for you. One is the cancer may pose very little danger because it will grow very slowly. That means you are far more likely to die from something other than prostate cancer. A second reason is it allows you to avoid the risk of getting any of the side effects that might occur when the prostate gland is treated. By not doing anything to the prostate, you are able to maintain your current quality-of-life until it changes due to aging. For example, surgery can cause immediate impotence that may last for the rest of your life. With watchful waiting, impotence may never occur or it may not happen until you are much older. Until then, you are able to keep having erections.

There is a risk with watchful waiting. By not treating your cancer, you might miss out on a chance to be cured. Some men feel that they would be willing to get treated when the cancer begins to cause a problem. By that time, however, it is more likely to be growing outside of the prostate, which is harder to cure. Another risk is the possibility that delaying treatment might allow the cancer to spread to other parts of your body. That could affect your quality-of-life and may shorten your survival.

What Are the Outcomes With Watchful Waiting?

You can get a good idea of what happens with watchful waiting by reviewing the results from several studies. The best one is a randomized study that compared it to radical prostatectomy. Men up to age 75 were eligible but the average age was 65. After five years, the percentage of men dying from prostate cancer or getting metastatic disease was the same in both groups. At 10 years, the percentage of men dying from prostate cancer was 5% higher in the watchful waiting group. The following table shows more recent results with longer follow-up.

Outcome After 12 Years	Watchful Waiting	Radical Prostatectomy
Alive	60.2%	67.3%
Died from prostate cancer	17.9%	12.5%
Died from other causes	21.9%	21.2%
Developed metastatic disease	26%	19.3%

At 12 years, surgery prevented 5.4% of the men from dying of prostate cancer. That means one person avoided dying out of every 18 who had surgery. It also prevented 1 out of every 15 men from getting metastatic disease. This study found that the age of the men greatly affected the results. Those men younger than 65 had an 18% lower chance of dying from their disease compared to the men of the same age on watchful waiting. That means surgery helped almost one out of every six younger men. Older men having the operation were just as likely to die as the men on watchful waiting. The study is continuing so the results could change with longer follow-up.

Another result from not doing surgery is the cancer can grow. This is called *local progression*. In some cases, it can cause men to have problems urinating or having a bowel movement. By 12 years, local progression occurred in 22% of men having surgery compared to 46% of men on watchful waiting. That means surgery prevented local progression in one out of every four men.

Local progression is far less of a problem to treat than metastatic prostate cancer. If you develop urinary difficulties during watchful waiting, it usually can be treated either with medication or a minor surgical procedure. Neither of them has the same risks as the treatments for prostate cancer. Occasionally, they are not sufficient to get rid of the symptoms. In those cases, radiation or hormone therapy can be used to shrink the prostate and improve urination.

Although this study was well designed, it does have some weaknesses.

- Some men assigned to get watchful waiting chose instead to have surgery.

- Some men assigned to get surgery refused to do it.

This happens in nearly every randomized study; some participants refuse to accept their assigned treatment. Doctors call a study "contaminated" when this occurs. In some cases, the contamination can be so high that the study becomes invalid. The contamination in this study is thought to be acceptable. Still, some doctors believe that surgery would have shown an even greater benefit if all the men had received their assigned treatment.

Because this is the only well-done study comparing these two treatments, many people want to use it for counseling men in the United States. One problem is this study included many men with more aggressive cancers than are found in the United States. Many doctors believe that surgery would show less benefit if a similar study was done in this country. The reasons are the following:

- More than 75% of the men in the study had stage T2 cancer but more than 60% of men in the United States have stage T1c.

- More than 50% of those in the study had a prostate-specific antigen (PSA) level greater than 10 ng/mL but more than 50% of men in the United States have a PSA level lower than 6.7 ng/mL.

- About 48% of men in the study had a Gleason score of 7 to 10 but more than 60% of men in the United States have a Gleason score of 6.

Despite the weaknesses, this is the only good study that compares watchful waiting to any other treatment. It shows that men on watchful waiting have a slightly higher risk of dying and getting metastatic disease compared to men getting a radical prostatectomy. In addition, men younger than 65 appear to have a large benefit from surgery but older men have almost none.

How Does Watchful Waiting Affect Your Quality-of-Life?

Another study was done on these same patients to determine the effect of surgery and watchful waiting on men's quality-of-life. Written surveys asking about sexual and urinary function were mailed to nearly one half of the men and were completed about four years after the study began. The results are shown in the next two tables.

Effect of Watchful Waiting or Surgery on Sexual Function

Survey Question	Watchful Waiting Group	Surgery Group
1. Erections seldom or never good enough for intercourse	45%	80%
2. Unable to maintain erections in more than one of every five attempts	30%	55%
3. No orgasm in the past six months	31%	62%

Effect of Watchful Waiting or Surgery on Urinary Function

Survey Question	Watchful Waiting Group	Surgery Group
1. Urinary stream weak more than one of every five times	44%	28%
2. Urinating at least twice per night	57%	44%
3. Leaking urine at least once per week	21%	49%
4. Moderate or severe distress from urinary leakage	9%	29%
5. Regular use of some protective aid for leakage	10%	43%

These tables show several key differences between the two groups. Compared to watchful waiting, more men treated with surgery are experiencing the following:

- Unable to achieve erections good enough for intercourse

- Unable to have an orgasm

- Unable to maintain an erection in at least one out of five attempts

- More likely to leak urine at least once per week

- Moderately or severely distressed by their leakage

The trade-off is that more men treated with watchful waiting experience the following:

- Have local progression of their cancer

- Get up at least twice per night to urinate

- Have a slow or weak urine stream

The erection problems that occurred for some of the men in the surgery group could be due to their also receiving hormone therapy rather than just having their prostate removed. That treatment can reduce erections.

This study also has some weaknesses.

- No baseline survey was done. Without that information, it is not possible to know if the sexual or urinary difficulties developed because men got older or they already were present when the study began. One thing is clear. Both problems may occur in some men as they get older but they are much more likely to occur following surgery.

- Only one half of the men who were in the study were sent the survey. One cannot assume that the same results would occur if all the men were surveyed.

- Surveys were completed by about 90% of the men who received one. It is not known how the results would be affected if the remaining 10% had answered the survey.

- Some men did not answer all the questions for unknown reasons.

- Twenty percent of the men assigned to have surgery did not get it yet they were still counted as if they had surgery. That may have underestimated the side effects in the surgery group.

- Six percent of the men in the watchful waiting group had surgery. They still were counted as if they had watchful waiting. That may have overestimated the side effects in the watchful waiting group.

- It is not known how many men had nerve-sparing surgery. A man will not have erections unless his nerves are preserved. Some of the men with stage T2 disease most likely had one or both nerves removed to avoid leaving cancer behind. This would increase their chances of having problems getting erections. Fewer men might have become impotent if a nerve-sparing operation had been done.

A radical prostatectomy has some other bothersome side effects that were not measured in this study but are shown in the next table. Their frequency has not been studied very well but they appear to occur in at least 10% of patients. They are explained in more detail in Chapter 11 on radical prostatectomy.

Other Side Effects of Radical Prostatectomy	Percentage of Patients
Hernias	3–10%
Shortening of the penis	50–80%
Painful orgasm	10–15%

Although this study reported short-term side effects, it did not include any longer-term quality-of-life results for the men who developed metastatic disease. The cancer and the treatment for it can greatly affect how men feel. The major side effects of treatment are shown in the following table and are further explained in Chapter 25.

Side Effects of Disease or Treatment of Metastatic Disease	Percentage of Patients
Bone pain	20–33%
Weight gain	3%
Bone fracture	6–9%
Hot flashes	21–73%
Decreased sex drive	40–60%
Decreased blood counts	90%
Urinary difficulties requiring surgery	10–25%

Side Effects of Disease or Treatment of Metastatic Disease	Percentage of Patients
Decreased energy	2–18%
Loss of appetite	
Impaired mental health	45–70%

Not included in this survey is the quality-of-life for the men who developed metastatic disease. The bottom line is neither report from the Swedish study was perfect. Nevertheless, *it is the only randomized study* ever done that included men treated with watchful waiting. It gives you some idea of the risks and benefits of this treatment.

Two other lesser quality studies provide additional information about watchful waiting. The first one was a retrospective study of men in Connecticut with clinical stage T1a, T1b, or T2 disease treated by watchful waiting between 1971 and 1982. It did not include men with stage T1c because the PSA test was not available at that time. Everyone was between the ages of 55 and 74 when their cancer was detected but the results have been divided into 5-year age groups according to the Gleason score on each biopsy. The results for the men diagnosed between the ages of 60 and 64 with a Gleason score of 6 are shown in next table. The study also contains results for men with other ages and Gleason scores.

Men Treated by Watchful Waiting

Outcome	At 5 Years	At 10 Years	At 15 Years	At 20 Years
Alive	85%	62%	42%	28%
Died of prostate cancer	5%	10%	20%	24%
Died of other causes	10%	28%	38%	48%

In this age group of men, the risk of dying from prostate cancer was approximately 10% by 10 years and 20% by 15 years after diagnosis. This study has strengths and weaknesses. Its weaknesses are the following:

- It is retrospective.

- The men were diagnosed more than 25 years ago.

- There could be a selection bias because men chose their treatment rather than being assigned to it.

- The results underestimate the risk of dying from prostate cancer because the average life expectancy is higher today than when the study was done.

Other doctors think the information is still very useful even today. They argue that men choosing watchful waiting today are more likely to live longer than those in the study for the following reasons:

- The survival has increased for men with advanced disease.

- Most cancers are diagnosed by the PSA test, which finds cancers that are less advanced. They progress more slowly and are less likely to be harmful over the next 10 years.

- More than 20% of the men did not have tests to determine whether the cancer had spread. If some of those men did not have localized disease, they would die sooner making the results look worse.

The bottom line is the results from this study provide some useful information about watchful waiting for men diagnosed today with clinical stage T1a, T1b, or T2 disease.

The last study also was retrospective but it includes men diagnosed by PSA testing (stage T1c) who were at least 65 years old. The cancers were found between 1992 and 2002 and were selected from Medicare patients located in four regions of the United States. The following table shows the patient's chance of dying from prostate cancer for different clinical stages, Gleason scores, and their age at diagnosis.

Percentage of Men on Watchful Waiting Who Died From Prostate Cancer in 10 Years

Clinical Tumor Stage When Diagnosed	Gleason Score	Age 65–69 at Diagnosis	Age 70–74 at Diagnosis	Age 75–79 at Diagnosis	Older Than Age 80 at Diagnosis
T1a or T1b	5, 6, or 7	Not enough men	3%	4%	6%
T1c	5, 6, or 7	2%	3%	6%	6%
T2	5, 6, or 7	7%	6%	8%	10%
T1a or T1b	8, 9, or 10	28%	25%	28%	29%
T1c	8, 9, or 10	9%	20%	17%	16%
T2	8, 9, or 10	29%	18%	22%	20%

This study shows that men older than the age of 65 with a Gleason score of 5, 6, or 7 have a low risk of dying from prostate cancer in 10 years. For those diagnosed by PSA testing, which is stage T1c, it happened to only 2% of men between the ages of 65 and 69. If they were older than the age of 80, only 6% died of their disease. This study also has strengths and weaknesses. The strengths are the following:

- It is the best information available about watchful waiting in men detected by PSA.

- It allows men to see what to expect based on their clinical stage.

The weaknesses are as follows:

- The study was retrospective. This means that there could be a bias in how men ended up with this therapy, they could have been less healthy, and some of the information could have been recorded incorrectly.

- It does not show what happens after 10 years. Longer follow-up might result in more cancer deaths.

- It combined the results for Gleason scores of 5, 6, and 7. A Gleason score of 7 is more dangerous than a Gleason score of 5 or 6. This means combining all three together will underestimate the risk of dying for men with a Gleason score of 7 but overestimate the risk for those with a Gleason score of 5 or 6.

- Men younger than the age of 65 were not included so younger men diagnosed with prostate cancer cannot assume they would get the same results from watchful waiting even if they have the same stage and Gleason score.

- The group with T1c tumors study was contaminated because nearly one quarter of them eventually had either surgery or radiation therapy. This could be making the results look better, which means the risk of dying may be underestimated.

Who Is a Good Candidate for Watchful Waiting?

Watchful waiting may be a very appropriate treatment for some men. The best candidates include the following:

- Most men older than age 75

- Men with major illnesses such as bad heart disease

- Men with a life expectancy of less than 10 years

- Men with low-risk disease, which means having a Gleason score of 6, a PSA level lower than 10 ng/mL, and a T1 or T2 cancer based on the digital rectal examination (DRE)

Watchful waiting is a bad choice for someone who has a Gleason score of 8, 9, or 10 even if his life expectancy is only five years. Those tumors are highly likely to progress and cause harm. Additionally, this would not be a good treatment if you are very anxious and will constantly worry about what is happening to your cancer.

How Will You Be Monitored on Watchful Waiting?

Before the PSA test was available, men were checked using the DRE and an annual bone scan. Today, most men on watchful waiting will have a DRE and PSA test done every 6 or 12 months. The bone scan does not need to be performed until the PSA level is more than 10 ng/mL or bone pain occurs because bone metastases are very uncommon at lower levels.

Many doctors also use the *PSA doubling time* as a basis for deciding when to do a bone scan. The doubling time is a measure of how long it takes for the PSA level to double in value. Good studies show that more than two thirds of men being diagnosed today have a PSA doubling time of more than four years. Because those tumors progress very slowly, doing a bone scan makes little sense unless the doubling time is closer to two years or less. If you want to know your PSA doubling time, two free tools are available for calculating it (http://kevin.phys.unm.edu/psa/ and http://www.mskcc.org/applications/nomograms/Prostate/PsaDoublingTime.aspx).

Suppose you have a bone scan and it is negative. When should it be done again? Most doctors will make the decision based on how fast the PSA level rises.

The Bottom Line About Watchful Waiting

Watchful waiting is the most conservative treatment for localized prostate cancer. It will result in the lowest chance of altering your quality-of-life right now and preserve it for many years. The trade-off is you have a slightly higher chance of dying or suffering from prostate cancer in the next 12 years. That risk is higher if you are young.

Around the United States, an increasing number of physicians are recognizing that many men are getting overtreated for prostate cancer. That has been the mixed blessing of PSA testing. Finding cancer earlier has made it easier to cure a man of his cancer, but it also has resulted in many men getting an unnecessary treatment for a cancer that never would have caused any harm. This chapter has given you a better idea of the risk posed by your cancer and what can happen to you if you choose watchful waiting. It should help you decide whether this is the right treatment for you.

Active Surveillance: A Safer Approach Than Watchful Waiting

10

What Is Active Surveillance?

It should be clear from the previous chapter that watchful waiting poses very little risk for many men. However, even a small risk is a gamble you may not be able or willing to accept. Also, the prospect of spending part of every day or week wondering if prostate cancer cells are spreading may cause you too much anxiety. Perhaps you might struggle with considerable guilt knowing you may have missed out on a chance to be cured. Living with those thoughts could worsen you and your family's quality-of-life.

Fortunately, there now is another approach. It is called *active surveillance* or *delayed therapy*. It differs from watchful waiting in that local treatment is delayed until there is some proof the cancer is dangerous. If nothing changes, active surveillance continues. If it does begin to grow or change, then active surveillance stops and local treatment is done.

The main advantage of active surveillance is it gives you a chance to avoid getting a treatment you never would have needed, which means you also avoid all potential side effects of that treatment. Active surveillance offers you a way to maintain your quality-of-life without the same risks that occur with watchful waiting. That means having the same sexual function and urinary control that existed before your diagnosis. The key to active surveillance is being able to tell when your cancer needs treatment before it becomes incurable.

Active surveillance does have some risk. Today, most newly diagnosed cancers can be cured because all the cancer cells are inside the prostate gland. Delaying treatment gives the tumor time to spread, making it harder to cure and increasing the chance it will recur. That could result in a decreased quality-of-life and a shortened survival.

What Are the Results With Active Surveillance?

Active surveillance is a relatively new way to treat men with localized prostate cancer. So far, few studies have been published and only one has followed men for more than 10 years. It is a prospective cohort study that began in Canada in 1995. The study has enrolled over 450 men, of which more than one half were younger than the age of 71. Most of the men had "low-risk" prostate cancer, which is a Gleason score of 6, a prostate-specific antigen (PSA) level of up to 10 ng/mL, and a tumor stage of T1 or T2a. The others had "intermediate" risk tumors that included either a PSA level of more than 10 ng/mL, a Gleason score of 7, or stage T2b or T2c disease. About one half of the group has been followed for at least seven years, but only a few men have been followed for 15 years.

All the men had a PSA measured every three months for two years and then every six months. A biopsy was done between 6 and 12 months after diagnosis and then every three years until age 80. Treatment was recommended for any one of the following reasons.

- The PSA level doubled in less than three years.

- The Gleason score increased.

- The tumor felt larger on the digital rectal examination (DRE).

The key *estimated* results from this study are shown in the following table.

Estimated Results of Active Surveillance

Outcome	Total at 5 Years	Total at 10 Years
Overall survival	90% (range 87%–93%)	68% (range 62%–74%)
Died from prostate cancer	0.3%	2.8%
Stayed on active surveillance	72%	62%
PSA progression after surgery or radiation in men stopping active surveillance	53%	Not available

Although many men have not been followed for a full 5 and 10 years, the estimated range of results is very narrow. That means the survival rate at 10 years could be as low as 62% or as high as 74%. There is no way to be more exact. So far, more than 60% of the group remains on active surveillance while 30% were advised to get treated. Also, only 3% have died from prostate cancer and 13% had a rise in PSA level within 10 years of their diagnosis.

The study has both strengths and weaknesses. It was a prospective cohort study that provides better information than retrospective studies (see Chapter 7). However, because it did not assign men to this treatment, there could be some selection bias. Perhaps some men chose active surveillance because they were less healthy. That would mean they are more likely to die of other causes than men getting another treatment. This would make the results appear more favorable.

Another possible bias is that these men had less cancer than those who choose immediate surgery or radiation. Both of these might make the results look better. Lastly, the impact of this treatment on men's quality-of-life has not been reported.

Comparing Active Surveillance and Radical Prostatectomy

Comparing the results from this study with other treatments is difficult because the patients may have different characteristics. Only randomized studies can accurately compare results. Without them, the best that can be done is to compare results from other studies that *seem* to have similar patients. Using that approach, the odds of being alive at 10 years following active surveillance or radical prostatectomy are very similar.

According to this study, active surveillance enables 70% of the men to avoid getting their prostate treated. Of the remaining 30% who did get a delayed treatment, about one half of them had a rise in their PSA level in 10 years. Is active surveillance as good as radical prostatectomy? That question cannot be answered reliably without a properly done study.

Who Is a Good Candidate for Active Surveillance?

At this time, no one can be sure who is an ideal candidate for active surveillance. Most doctors believe that if you have a Gleason score of 8, 9, or 10 on your biopsy, then this is not the right treatment unless your life expectancy is less than five years. The following chart shows the different requirements being used to select men for active surveillance in the United States.

Best Candidates for Active Surveillance

---

1. Clinical stage T1c or T2a

2. PSA level of less than 10 ng/mL

3. Gleason score of 3 + 3 = 6

4. If older than the age of 70: Gleason score of 3 + 4 = 7 or PSA level up to 15 ng/mL

Best Candidates for Active Surveillance (Continued)

5. Cancer cells found on less than three cores

6. Cancer cells found in less than 50% of any one core

7. PSA doubling time greater than three years

This list may change as more studies report their results.

How Will I Be Followed on Active Surveillance?

Because active surveillance is so new, the best way to check you is still being worked out. So far, the time it takes for the PSA level to double, the DRE and the results found on repeat prostate biopsies are being used to determine when active surveillance should be stopped. A PSA test and a DRE are being performed every three to six months, and a biopsy is being done annually or at 1, 2, and 5 years after diagnosis. Between 8 and 12 cores are being done for the repeat biopsies. Research is in progress to find other ways to tell if you need treatment. For now, staying on active surveillance is okay if you satisfy the following characteristics.

Requirements for Remaining on Active Surveillance

1. The time it takes for your PSA level to double must be longer than three years.

2. The biopsy cannot show more cancer cells than the previous biopsy.

3. The Gleason score must remain stable or decrease.

4. Your prostate exam cannot show an increase in the size of the tumor.

What Do Doctor Groups Say About Active Surveillance?

The American Urological Association (AUA) is the governing body for urologists in the United States. In 2008, they updated their guidelines for managing prostate cancer with the following statement:

- The three usual treatments for localized prostate cancer are active surveillance, radiation therapy and surgery. There is no information that shows one treatment is clearly better than the others.

The National Comprehensive Cancer Network (NCCN) is a group of doctors selected from major cancer centers in the United States. In 2010 they made the following statements about active surveillance for localized prostate cancer:

- Men with "low risk" prostate cancer who have a life expectancy of less than 10 years should be offered and recommended active surveillance. Patients with a low risk cancer include those with a stage T1 to T2a tumor, a Gleason score less than 7, and a PSA level below 10 ng/mL.

- Men with "very low risk" prostate cancer and a life expectancy of less than 20 years *should only be treated with active surveillance.* This includes men with:

A stage T1a tumor, a Gleason score less than 7 and a PSA level below 10 ng/mL

A biopsy showing less than three positive biopsy cores with cancer present in less than 50% of the sample.

A PSA density below 0.15 ng/mL per gram. The PSA density is determined by dividing the PSA level by the size of the prostate as determined from a prostate ultrasound.

You should be aware that this advice is *based only on the opinions* of those doctors on the panel and not on any good studies. At this time, no one knows what will happen to men who are on active surveillance for 15 years or longer.

The Bottom Line About Active Surveillance

Contrary to initial fears, active surveillance with delayed treatment has not resulted in a high risk of dying from prostate cancer in 5 and 10 years. It has enabled more than 60% of men to avoid a treatment that so far would have been unnecessary. It offers you a way to make sure that treatment really is needed. Although there is a chance that your cancer might be incurable by the time it is treated, so far, the chances of that occurring are very low. Also, the risk of dying from prostate cancer in 10 years is very low. However, you are more likely to get a rise in your PSA level in 10 years if treatment is delayed. More information is needed to tell you what to expect from active surveillance beyond 10 years. At this time, no one can say whether this treatment is as good, better, or worse than getting therapy right away. Until a proper study is done, you may find this approach to be an appealing alternative to immediate treatment or watchful waiting. Only you can decide if the risks are worth the benefits. At the very least, your doctor should discuss active surveillance as one of the options for managing localized prostate cancer.

Surgical Treatment of Localized Prostate Cancer

Of all the treatments available for localized prostate cancer, *radical prostatectomy* has been in use for the longest time and has the longest follow-up information. For that reason, many doctors call it the "the gold standard." It is called a "radical" prostatectomy because the entire prostate is removed along with both seminal vesicles and a portion of both vas deferens (see Chapter 4).

One of the most important advances in this operation was the discovery of how to remove the entire prostate without injuring the two *pelvic nerves* that enable men to have erections. This operation is called a *nerve-sparing radical prostatectomy*, and it has had a huge impact on men's quality-of-life. There are many things you should know about the radical prostatectomy before deciding if it is the right treatment for you.

What Are the Advantages and Disadvantages of a Radical Prostatectomy?

The advantage of removing the prostate is that it *may* immediately remove all the cancer in your body, meaning you *may* never have a problem from prostate cancer in the future. In other words, you *may* be cured.

The reason for saying "may" rather than "will" is that radical prostatectomy does not cure everyone. Sometimes, cancer cells already may be in the surrounding tissues or in other parts of the body. The operation does not remove those cells and they may continue to grow, causing problems in the future. A second problem is the operation may cause side effects or complications that affect your quality-of-life. Lastly, you could get an unnecessary treatment because your cancer would never have harmed you as was explained in Chapter 9.

What Are the Results With Radical Prostatectomy?

Only one good study has been done comparing radical prostatectomy to any other option, in this case to watchful waiting. It was reviewed in Chapter 9 and showed that radical prostatectomy reduced the chance of cancer spreading and increased survival, but it only helped about 1 out of every 15 men in 10 years. This study has some weaknesses, but it is the best information available. The conclusion is that taking out the prostate is better for controlling prostate cancer than just watching it.

Is surgery better than the other treatments for prostate cancer? The answer is not clear because doctors now realize that not all prostate tumors behave the same. They can be divided into low-risk, intermediate-risk, and high-risk. Each has a different chance of causing harm. Without good studies like the one discussed earlier, the best that can be said is *the 10-year results of radical prostatectomy appear to be similar to external radiation and brachytherapy.* Not enough information is available about the other treatment options for them to be compared.

What Are the Potential Complications of Radical Prostatectomy?

In the past, a radical prostatectomy was associated with a high complication rate. Fortunately, surgeons have found ways to make the operation much safer. The complications can be divided into short term and long term; short term means they happen in the first 30 days after surgery, and long term is anything beyond that time. The odds of them occurring depend on many things including the quality of your surgeon, your age and health, and your prostate cancer. Still, the results give you some idea of the risks associated with this treatment. Many of the studies are several years old so the complication rates may be lower in men having surgery now.

Short-term Complications After Radical Prostatectomy

Complication	Approximate Frequency (%)
1. Infection	1.6%–1.9%
2. Bleeding requiring transfusion	3% (for laparoscopic, robotic) 2–21% (for retropubic)
3. Deep venous thrombosis	1%–2%
4. Injury to rectum requiring colostomy	Less than 1%
5. Injury to internal organ	Less than 0.5%
6. Lymphocele	2%–4%
7. Pulmonary embolus	1%–2%
8. Respiratory problems	4%–7%
9. Heart attack, congestive heart failure	2%–3%
10. Death	0.1%–0.2%

Explanation of Side Effects and How They Are Treated

Infections can occur either in the urine, on the skin where the surgeon made a cut, or deep inside the pelvis near the prostate. The first two can be treated with antibiotics. The third one may be caused by a fluid collection called an *abscess*, which is treated with antibiotics and by draining or removing the fluid. Usually, this can be done by inserting a needle through the skin and using an x-ray to guide it into the abscess. The fluid is taken out by attaching a syringe to the needle. On rare occasions, a patient may have to return to the operating room to have the wound reopened and the infection be drained.

Deep venous thrombosis or DVT—a blood clot that forms in a leg vein. It is treated in the hospital with *anticoagulants* to "thin the blood." Sometimes the blood clot moves to the lung forming a *pulmonary embolus* (PE), which can be life threatening. It also is treated with blood thinners, but surgery might be needed to remove the clot.

Colostomy—an opening into the rectum may occur during the operation because the rectum is next to the prostate. Depending on its size, the surgeon may be able to close it with a few stitches. Sometimes the bowel must be cut and brought to the skin to allow the injury to heal. This is called a *colostomy*. A special bag is kept on the skin to collect the bowel contents. Six weeks later, another operation is done to close the colostomy.

Injuries—injuries to other internal organs include an artery, vein, the bladder, or the *ureter*, which is the tube that carries urine from the kidney to the bladder. All these injuries can be repaired during the prostatectomy, providing the surgeon knows it occurred. On rare occasions, these injuries are not found until sometime after surgery and then another operation may be needed to correct the problem.

Lymphocele—when lymph nodes are removed, lymph sometimes leaks into the surrounding tissues and forms a fluid collection. It can cause pain and fever, which must be drained. In most cases, an x-ray can be used to guide a needle through the skin and into the exact site to drain the fluid.

Respiratory problems—all operations have the potential to cause respiratory problems such as pneumonia. They usually respond to antibiotics.

Heart attack, congestive heart failure, and death—all of these can also occur with any operation. A heart attack and congestive heart failure require hospitalization.

Long-term Complications Following Radical Prostatectomy

Complications	Odds They May Occur
Leaking urine (urinary incontinence)	3%–30%
Difficulty having erections (impotence)	20%–90%
Urethral stricture	5%–14%
Inguinal hernia	3%–10%
Penile shortening	50%–80%
Pain during ejaculation	10%–15%
Dry orgasm	100%

Urinary incontinence—this means urine leaks out from the penis. It can vary from a few drops with heavy exertion to leaking urine every minute of the day. Urinary incontinence probably is the most embarrassing side effect of radical prostatectomy. It happens to almost every man immediately after surgery. Some improve very quickly although others take up to a year to fully regain control. A small percentage never get back to normal and require either medication, the use of pads inside their underwear, or even surgery to correct the problem.

Impotence—means being unable to have an erection good enough for sexual intercourse. Even when a nerve-sparing prostatectomy is done properly, some men become impotent for reasons doctors cannot explain. Most men having surgery do not regain their ability to have erections for several months, but it can take up to two years.

Urethral stricture—a scar that forms in the tube carrying urine from the bladder out through the tip of the penis. A urethral stricture can be *dilated* using a rubber or metal instrument passed into the penis and through the scar. Another option is to cut the scar by placing an instrument with an attached knife into the urethra. It is done under some type of anesthesia and is completed in less than 15 minutes. Occasionally, these treatments can result in more urinary leakage, which may be permanent. Urethral strictures can recur.

Inguinal hernia—an extension of a portion of the intestine down toward the scrotum. It feels like a bulge in the groin area. This has not been widely recognized as a side effect of a radical prostatectomy, but several good studies have shown that it does occur. Doctors think that some men have an undiscovered hernia that is made worse by the operation. The frequency of hernias is not increased in men having a perineal prostatectomy. A hernia can be detected by examination before surgery but most doctors don't do it. If you are planning to have this treatment, you should ask your doctor to examine you while standing and straining. This is called a *valsalva maneuver*. If a hernia is found, it can be fixed during the prostatectomy. Otherwise, another operation will be needed.

Penile shortening—this is another side effect not often discussed with patients but it happens in most men. The loss is greatest within a few weeks of surgery and gets better after a year. Even at that time, men may lose 0.5 to 4 cm of the length of the penis. There is no proven treatment for it at this time but doctors are exploring ways to help this problem.

Painful orgasm—another side effect seldom discussed by surgeons. It usually lasts for about one minute. Some men report it's so severe that it interferes with normal sexual function. Studies have not been done to know the best way to treat it.

Dry orgasm—during the operation, the tubes carrying seminal fluid to the penis are cut, preventing any fluid from coming out. A dry orgasm will be permanent, and there is no treatment for it. Some men report this decreases their pleasure during sexual activity. When this occurs, men are unable to father a child by having intercourse.

By now, you might be overwhelmed as you read about all these side effects and the odds they might occur. As you discuss this treatment with your doctor, one of the key questions to get answered is, "What are my odds of getting all three of the major results; being free of my cancer, eventually getting complete control of my urine and having sexual function return to where it started?" Some people called it the "trifecta" result. No one can predict what will definitely happen to you but at least you now have some idea of the odds these side effects might occur.

Who Is a Good Candidate for Radical Prostatectomy?

Most doctors believe that any man with localized prostate cancer who is likely to live at least 10 or 15 years is a good candidate for this treatment. The reason for putting those numbers on life expectancy is that most prostate cancers diagnosed today will not grow very fast. Even if left untreated, they will not cause problems for at least 10 years. The exception is men with a Gleason score above 7. They are much more dangerous. About 20% of them will die from their disease within five years of diagnosis if they are not treated. They might benefit from surgery if their life expectancy is at least five years.

Which Operation Is Right for You?

The first radical prostatectomy was performed more than 60 years ago by making a cut in the skin from below the belly button down to the pubic bone. This is called a *radical retropubic prostatectomy* or RRP. Three other methods are now available:

- *radical perineal prostatectomy* (RPP)

- *laparoscopic radical prostatectomy* (LRP)

- *robot-assisted laparoscopic radical prostatectomy* (RALP)

A nerve sparing radical prostatectomy can be done using any of the four methods.

So, which method should you have? If you read the commercials on billboards or Web sites, you would think that the robotic-assisted method is the only way to go. But the facts are that each method has potential advantages and disadvantages. No good study has ever proven that one of them does a better job of controlling the cancer, causing less urinary leakage or fewer problems with erections. For that reason, they are all equally good choices for removing your prostate.

What about recovering from surgery, is one better than another? One randomized study showed no difference in pain during the first 14 days between the retropubic and robotic methods. Two definite differences are that the retropubic prostatectomy has more blood loss and more men get blood transfusions. Uncontrolled studies show similar complication rates with all four methods. The only major factor that seems to influence the results is the experience of the surgeon. That means the most important question for you to answer is "who should do your operation?" rather than "how should it be done?"

Should You Get Hormone Therapy Before Surgery?

Because not every man will be cured by surgery, doctors have asked if anything can be done to improve the results. One option is to lower the male hormone called *testosterone* for several months because that can kill prostate cancer cells. One name for this treatment is *hormone therapy*, and it is explained in detail in Chapter 25. Several good quality studies have tested this idea in men scheduled for surgery, and none of them found an improvement in survival or a lowering of the chance of getting a recurrence. Therefore, *hormone therapy should not be done* even if your surgery is delayed for several months. It actually could make the operation more difficult and make you lose more blood. Despite these studies, some doctors still do it. If your doctor wants you to get this treatment, you should either ask how it will help you or consider getting a second opinion.

What Happens Before the Operation?

Regardless of how the prostate will be removed, you first must have a preoperative evaluation that is done about one or two weeks before the operation. A complete physical examination and a heart test called an *electrocardiogram* or *ECG* will be performed. Blood will be taken to measure your blood count, called a *complete blood count* (CBC), and the amount of *sodium, potassium, chloride, carbon dioxide, blood urea nitrogen,* and *glucose* in the bloodstream. Additional tests may be ordered depending on your medical history. The goal of these tests is to make sure nothing is wrong that might increase your risk of having complications after the operation.

For at least one week before surgery, you should not take over-the-counter medications that can increase your risk of bleeding. That includes any drug belonging to a group called *nonsteroidal anti-inflammatory drugs* or *NSAIDs* such as aspirin, Motrin, ibuprofen, Naprosyn, Aleve, and Celebrex. Vitamin E also should be avoided for the same reason. If one of these is taken by mistake within seven days of surgery, your doctor should be notified right away. You should not eat or drink anything after midnight of the evening before surgery.

What to Expect the Day of Surgery

You will be told to arrive at the hospital or surgical center a few hours before the scheduled time of the operation. Once there, you will change into a surgical gown and then be placed on a cart. Some surgeons doing a retropubic prostatectomy will ask that a blood sample be sent to the blood bank to cross-match blood in case it is needed. An intravenous line is inserted into your arm to administer fluids and medications. You may receive a drug to relax you before being taken into the operating room.

A radical prostatectomy is performed under *general* or *spinal anesthesia*. General anesthesia means you are put to sleep and usually a tube is placed down your windpipe through your mouth. A ventilator will control your breathing and deliver a gas that keeps you asleep.

Spinal anesthesia means you are awake but you will be unable to feel any pain in the lower half of your body. You still will breath on your own. The spinal anesthesia is done by inserting a small needle into your lower back and injecting the anesthetic drugs into the fluid surrounding your spinal cord. During the surgery, the anesthesiologist can give you other medication to make you sleepy so you don't have to listen to the sounds in the operating room. The perineal, laparoscopic, and robot-assisted laparoscopic operations usually are done under general anesthesia, and the retropubic approach can be done either way. After the anesthetic takes effect, the skin is washed and covered with an antiseptic solution, sterile drapes are placed over the surgical site, and then the operation can begin.

Radical Retropubic Prostatectomy

This operation takes about three hours to complete with you lying on your back on the operating table. The surgeon begins by cutting the skin from just below the belly button down to your pubic bone. The length of the incision varies depending on your height but is usually about 8 to 10 cm long. No muscles are cut; they are simply spread apart to allow the surgeon to reach your prostate.

One advantage of the retropubic approach over the laparoscopic and robotic methods is the ability to feel the prostate, the surrounding tissues, and the pelvic lymph nodes. This is important in some cases, because it helps the surgeon decide whether it is safe to do a nerve-sparing radical prostatectomy. After the prostate is exposed, the surface of the prostate is examined. If it feels smooth, the nerves can be saved because they probably are not invaded by cancer. However, if the surgeon feels a lump, hardness, or any other abnormality near the nerve, the safest approach is to take it out. If both nerves feel abnormal, then both should be removed. Of course, this is a very subjective evaluation. There is no completely accurate way to tell if cancer is present in a pelvic nerve without removing it.

There is another option if the surgeon is unsure about saving the nerves. They can be left in place, and a *frozen section* can be requested after the prostate is removed. This means the pathologist will immediately examine the tissue under a microscope to see if cancer has grown outside the prostate near the location of each nerve. If that has happened, then one or both nerves can be removed before the operation is over.

A second advantage of the retropubic approach is the ability to *feel* the lymph nodes, which is not possible with the other three methods. If a lymph node feels enlarged or hard, it could mean that prostate cancer has spread or *metastasized* to that lymph node. In that case, the surgeon can remove the lymph node and do a *frozen section biopsy* before taking out the prostate. The optimal management of patients who may have prostate cancer in the lymph nodes is discussed in the next chapter. Fortunately, your odds of having cancer in the lymph nodes probably are very low so this may not be a real advantage for you.

The retropubic approach does have some disadvantages compared to the other three methods. It results in more blood loss and a greater chance of needing a transfusion. The average amount is about 1,000 to 1,500 mL or about 4 or 5 pints (pt), but this is very dependent on the experience of the surgeon. Between 2% and 21% of men get a transfusion.

Because of the potential blood loss, many doctors have asked their patients to donate 1 or 2 pt of blood a few weeks before surgery. It is given back during or shortly after the operation. In recent years, this is done less often because banked blood is much safer now and less bleeding occurs. The approximate risks from getting banked blood are shown in the table.

Complications of Blood Transfusion	Frequency
Allergic reaction	1 out of every 333 pt
Hepatitis B	1 out of every 205,000 pt
Human immunodeficiency virus (HIV)	1 out of every 2,135,000 pt
Fever	1 out of every 100 pt

If you are going to have a retropubic prostatectomy, ask how often your doctor gives a transfusion and then decide if you want to donate your blood, accept blood from the blood bank, or choose a different surgeon. Donating your own blood is not necessarily a good thing to do because it will lower your blood count going into the operation. Combining the blood lost during surgery with a low blood count before starting the operation substantially raises the chances you will need a transfusion. A fever or other allergic reaction can happen even from receiving your own blood.

Another disadvantage of the retropubic approach is that the average hospital stay is one or two nights longer compared to the other methods. This, too, is dependent on your surgeon.

The last problem is that you have to wait about six weeks before resuming all physical activities compared to about three or four weeks with the other methods. If you would like to resume those activities as soon as possible, then you should find a surgeon who will use one of the other surgical approaches.

Radical Perineal Prostatectomy

The perineal approach is the least commonly performed radical prostatectomy in the United States because not many doctors have been trained to do it. This is unfortunate because it has very good results. It can be completed in one to two hours and is always performed using general anesthesia because you must be placed in the lithotomy position with your legs raised off the table. You would be too uncomfortable if you were awake during this operation.

After the rectal area is cleansed and coated with an antiseptic, the operation begins. The surgeon makes a curved cut in the skin underneath the scrotum in front of the rectum. The length of this cut is about 6 to 8 cm.

The perineal approach causes less blood loss than the retropubic method, rarely requiring a transfusion. That means you will not need to donate your blood. An advantage of the perineal operation compared to the laparoscopic and robot-assisted approach is that the surgeon can feel along the pelvic nerves to determine if they can be saved or must be removed. This operation usually takes less time to complete than the other methods. Another advantage is that the surgical scar will not be visible when wearing a bathing suit, which might be important to you. Lastly, the perineal prostatectomy is the least-costly operation, which might be a concern if you have a very large insurance deductible or no insurance at all.

One disadvantage of this approach compared to the retropubic prostatectomy is that the surgeon cannot feel the lymph nodes or remove them. Thus, the perineal approach should not be used if the risk of cancer in the lymph nodes is high (see Chapter 12). The bottom line is this method is a very good option when performed by an experienced surgeon.

Laparoscopic Radical Prostatectomy

The laparoscopic approach is often described by key words such as "minimally invasive," or "keyhole surgery" because it requires a smaller incision than with the retropubic approach. This operation takes about three hours to complete, although occasionally it may take much longer.

After the anesthetic is started, the abdomen is washed, coated with an antiseptic, and covered with sterile drapes. The operation begins by first inserting a needle into the abdomen and inflating it with carbon dioxide. This separates the abdominal wall from the internal organs, making a space to do the surgery. Three or four skin openings are made in the lower abdomen each about 5 to 10 mm in length. Surgical instruments and a telescopic lens are inserted through these openings and passed inside the body. A camera is connected to the lens, which shows the surgical area on a TV screen located in the operating room. The surgeon performs the operation by looking at the TV screen rather than at the patient. After the prostate has been cut away from the bladder and the urethra, a 4- to 6-cm incision is made above the pubic bone to remove the prostate from the body.

The laparoscopic approach first became popular after 2000, but the development of the robotic approach has resulted in it being done much less often. One disadvantage is it requires doing many cases before a surgeon gets good results. If your surgeon tells you that the laparoscopic approach will be used, be sure to ask *exactly* how many he or she has performed. If it is under 50 or 100, be aware that your risk for complications may be higher and the duration of your surgery may be longer compared to the other surgical methods or having a more experienced surgeon do it.

The laparoscopic approach does have the advantages of less blood loss and a slightly shorter time in the hospital compared to the retropubic approach. It is similar to the perineal and robotic methods. One disadvantage of the laparoscopic method is the inability to feel the nerves or the lymph nodes, although both can be removed by this operation. Another disadvantage is a slightly greater risk of injuring the bladder, bowel, or a blood vessel compared to the retropubic or perineal approach.

Robot-Assisted Laparoscopic Radical Prostatectomy

Beginning in approximately 2001, new developments in technology enabled surgeons to perform the laparoscopic operation with the assistance of a robotic device. The popularity of this approach has exploded due in part to good, but sometimes misleading advertising. The average RALP takes about three hours to complete, but occasionally, it can take much longer.

The operation starts in the same way as the laparoscopic prostatectomy. The anesthetic is started and the abdomen is washed, coated with an antiseptic, and draped. A needle is placed into the abdomen to inflate it with carbon dioxide then three or four cuts are made in the skin. Operating instruments and a telescopic lens are inserted through these openings and then robotic arms are attached to each of them. Special cables connect the robotic arms to instruments on another table several feet from the operating table. The surgeon sits at this table and looks through two eyepieces that give a three-dimensional view of the inside of the belly. Two robotic controls on the console are used to perform the operation; every movement by the surgeon results in an identical movement of the robotic arms connected to the patient. After the prostate has been separated from the bladder and urethra, it is removed by making a 4-cm cut in the skin. This method is easier to learn than the laparoscopic method perhaps because it gives a 3-dimensional view during the operation. Still, it may take over 50 or 100 cases to get good results so be sure to ask how many your surgeon has done.

The advantages of RALP are that it also has less blood loss, rarely requires a blood transfusion, and has a slightly shorter time in the hospital than the retropubic operation. These are the same advantages as the perineal and laparoscopic approach. Also, it does provide the surgeon with a bigger view of the surgical area than the retropubic or perineal methods. You may resume vigorous activities one to two weeks sooner than after the retropubic approach. The disadvantage of an RALP is that the surgeon cannot feel the lymph nodes or the pelvic nerves, which may be unimportant with most cancers diagnosed today.

Completing the Operation

The remainder of the operation is the same for all four methods. The surgeon will disconnect your prostate and seminal vesicles from the blood vessels, urethra, and the bladder, remove it from the body, and send it to the pathologist. After the prostate is out, the surgeon sews your bladder to the urethra. A rubber tube called a Foley catheter is inserted through the penis and passed into the bladder. It is left in place for 3 to 14 days to allow healing to occur. The duration of this catheter varies among surgeons.

The Foley catheter is held in place by a small water-filled balloon located at the end of the catheter sitting in the bladder. The other end is connected to a bag that collects the urine as it drains from your bladder. You will be taught how to disconnect the bag from the catheter and empty the bag when it is full. Two types of bags are used. A large one is used mostly at night so you don't have to get up to empty it. It lies on the floor or attaches to the lower part of the bed. You should always keep the bag below your bladder otherwise a urinary infection might occur. The smaller bag is used during the day. It straps to the leg and is hidden under your pants allowing you to walk around without people noticing it. It is emptied directly into the toilet.

Near the end of the operation, another rubber tube, called a surgical drain is placed near the connection between the bladder and urethra. Many doctors performing a laparoscopic or robotic-assisted prostatectomy have stopped doing using it. When it is used, the drain comes out of the body through a small opening made in the skin. It is located near the cut made to remove the prostate. The drain helps avoid an infection by removing any fluids that collect in the pelvis. It is held in place by a suture placed in the skin. The openings in the skin are closed either with staples or sutures depending on which surgical method was used.

What to Expect After the Operation

When the operation is over, you will be transferred to the recovery room and remain there until the anesthetic has worn off. Pain medication and intravenous fluids are given as needed. You will be transferred to a hospital bed when stable. Usually, you can begin drinking fluids and possibly begin eating later in the day or the following morning. The nurses will encourage you to cough and take breaths to avoid getting pneumonia. You can go home when you are able to eat, walk, have a normal temperature, your pain is controlled by pills, and there is no evidence of an infection. Before being discharged, the drain is removed by cutting the suture and slowly sliding it out through the opening in the skin. This causes very little discomfort and takes less than one minute. The drain site is then covered with a bandage, which you can change at home if needed.

What Happens After Leaving the Hospital?

Your doctor will advise you to wait one or two days before showering. After 5 to 10 days, you must return to have the wound checked and possibly the Foley catheter removed. The sutures used to close the incisions after the perineal, laparoscopic, and robotic operations are placed under the skin and will dissolve. The staples used to close the incision used for the retropubic operation will be removed during your visit. Some doctors perform an x-ray called a *cystogram* before taking out the catheter to make sure the connection between the bladder and urethra has healed. A dye is placed into the bladder through the catheter just before the x-ray is done. If a leak is seen, the catheter is left in place for another one or two weeks.

Before removing the Foley catheter, a syringe is attached to it to remove the fluid inside the balloon. The catheter then is slowly withdrawn, which takes less than two minutes and usually causes only minor discomfort. In most cases, urine leaks from the penis after the catheter is out. Bringing a pair of Depenz or some other absorbing material to wear underneath your clothes can avoid embarrassing leakage until you get home. Wearing dark colored pants are recommended because they hide any leakage that might occur.

The amount of leakage and how long it will last varies among patients. You can help yourself by doing *Kegel exercises*. The way to learn how to do them is to start to urinate while in the shower and then tighten the pelvic muscles until the urine flow stops. Good studies have shown that starting these exercises either four weeks before the operation or just after the catheter has been removed can shorten the time to recovery. It also can result in better urinary control one year after the operation. The following schedule was used in one study that showed these exercises were helpful:

- Alternate 10 contractions lasting 5 seconds with 10 seconds of muscular relaxation.

- Perform the exercises sitting, standing, squatting, and going up and down stairs.

- Perform three sets of exercises daily for six months.

Most doctors probably are not aware of these results so your best course of action is to begin these exercises on your own a few weeks before surgery. If you have leakage, most doctors will tell you to be patient because it takes time to improve. Some men regain complete control very quickly but up to one year may be required before the leakage stops completely. You can place an absorbent pad inside your underwear until the leakage stops. In some cases, the leakage may not completely disappear.

Another important part of your recovery is doing something to help your sexual function. Opinions vary on what to do. Most doctors have no specific advice although others suggest taking Viagra, Levitra, or Cialis on a regular basis or using a *vacuum pump* device. The options available for improving your sexual function are discussed in Chapter 19.

Follow-up Care

Most men begin to feel reasonably well within two weeks of surgery, but this is quite variable. Vigorous exercise or heavy lifting or straining should be avoided for two weeks following a perineal operation, four weeks after the robot-assisted or laparoscopic operation, and about six weeks after the retropubic operation. Most doctors have their patients return for an evaluation about every three months during the first year and every three to six months in the second year. At each visit, a prostate-specific antigen (PSA) and digital rectal exam (DRE) will be performed. Any decision about additional treatment will be made based on your pathology report from surgery and the PSA level. Even if you get a good result, you should continue to have a PSA yearly because the cancer can reappear many years later.

How Do You Choose a Surgeon?

Some studies have shown that surgeons who do more than 20 or 40 radical prostatectomies per year have fewer complications compared to less-experienced surgeons. The problem is that most urologists in the United States do not do that many. A survey in 2005 found that 80% of urologists perform no more than 10 of them per year.

So, how do you choose a surgeon? Should it be the urologist who found your cancer, another doctor in the community, or do you need to go to someone who specializes in performing this operation? Don't expect your urologist to volunteer to tell you how many they have done or refer you to someone else who might have more experience. But *if you want to have the best chance for a good result, have your surgery done by a very experienced surgeon.* Many cities have "specialists" that focus mostly on doing this operation. The only way to find out your doctor's experience is to ask, "How many of these operations do you do each year and how many have you done in your career?" Do not be afraid to do this because you have every right to know the answer and it is not your concern if their ego is hurt. You are the one who has to live with the results and that depends greatly on the surgeon's experience. Although doing less than 20 per year does not mean a surgeon gets worse results, it is one factor to consider.

Another way to choose your surgeon is to ask specific questions about complications. Too often, doctors will tell you the possible complications of the operation but they don't tell you how often they occur. Others will give you the results reported in medical journals. Keep in mind that the most experienced surgeons in the country write these papers, so if your doctor is not one of them, his or her results probably are not as good.

The following questions also can help you decide who should do your operation. Write them on a piece of paper and take them with you when you have a consultation regarding your treatment.

- What percentage of your patients with erections similar to mine is able to have intercourse without any aids 12 to 18 months after surgery?

- How many of them use aids such as medication or a pump?

- What percentage of your patients has the same urinary control one year after surgery as they did before the operation?

- What percentage of your patients develops other complications and how often does each one occur?

If you decide to ask any of these questions, you also should ask how your doctor got this information. Was it estimated or was a written survey used that has been shown to provide more accurate results? Asking patients during a follow-up visit, "How are you doing" or "Are you having any problems" *underestimates the complication rate.* The problem is that *very few* doctors routinely use these surveys, which means most do not know their true results. The best advice to give you is to choose a surgeon who uses a written survey, assuming you can find one nearby. If none is available in your community, at least choose a surgeon who has done many of these operations. The goal here is not be critical of your doctor but rather to help you get the right information so you can weigh the risks and benefits of this treatment.

Some surgeons may try to make you feel more comfortable by giving you the names of previously treated men to ask about their experience. The problem is that talking to someone with a "good" result really will not allow you to evaluate that doctor. In many ways, it is the same as the references you put on your own resume. Would you ever name someone who would not give you a good report? No, of course not! Still, you may find it helpful to ask a patient these questions.

- How long did you stay in the hospital?

- How long was the catheter left in your bladder?

- Was your pain well controlled after surgery?

- How was the nursing staff?

- What complications did you develop?

- How was the bedside manner of the physician?

- Was the doctor compassionate about your discomfort and feelings?

- Have you regained your urine control and sexual function and how long did it take?

- Did the doctor do a good job of explaining everything to you?

If you do decide to have a specialist perform your surgery, the next question is how do you find a good one? It may be necessary to call different doctors in your area to ask how many of these operations are done each year and how they assess their results. The best place to start is at a university hospital or a major medical institution. If none is nearby, consider going to another city. After you recover from your operation, a local doctor can do the follow-up care so you will not need constant travelling. You will be living a long time so it is worth a little inconvenience to get the best result possible.

Some men look for "Best Doctor Lists" published in books and magazines. You should know that these are more like popularity contests rather than a true measure of excellence. They are not based on any objective measurements such as cure rates or the percentage of men getting complications. Some doctors on those lists may not be that good, and doctors left off the list might be excellent.

What Are the Chances the Cancer Will Return?

After the prostate has been removed, the predominant source of PSA is gone so the PSA usually drops to less than 0.05 ng/mL. Because this takes about four weeks, measuring it before this time could give a falsely high number. Does a low PSA level mean you are cured? Not in all cases. A few cancer cells might still be in your body but they don't produce enough PSA to be detected by the test. Where would they be? Some could have grown into the area surrounding the prostate, some may have spread to other parts of the body, or some could be in multiple locations. As they divide, the PSA eventually will rise, which can take 15 years. That is why you should continue to have the test.

After your prostate is out, you might wonder about your odds of getting a recurrence. Fortunately, tools are available that can give you this information. One is called the *Kattan nomogram*, which is based on several characteristics about your tumor as shown in the following table.

Information Used for Kattan Nomogram

1. The PSA level before surgery.

2. The tumor stage before surgery.

3. The primary and secondary Gleason grade on the radical prostatectomy.

4. The extent of cancer in the prostate found at surgery.

5. The presence or absence of cancer in the seminal vesicles and lymph nodes.

This calculator is freely available at the Memorial Sloan Kettering Hospital Web site (http://www.mskcc.org). After entering the site, enter the type of cancer, which is prostate. Then click on "prostate cancer prediction tool" and select "prediction tool after radical prostatectomy." You can get all the information needed from a copy of your pathology report or from your doctor.

Primary and secondary Gleason grade: As explained in Chapter 6, every prostate cancer is given two numbers, each from one to five. It is based on how the cells appear when viewed under a microscope. The first number is called the *primary* Gleason grade. It is the number given to the most common type of cancer cells seen in the tissue. The second number is the *secondary* Gleason grade. It is the number given to the second most common type of cancer cells. Most operative reports provide these numbers. For example, a report may say, "Gleason score $3 + 3 = 6$ or $4 + 4 = 8$." If the report only gives the total Gleason score without the primary and secondary numbers, then you can contact the pathology department and ask for the individual numbers. If the Gleason score is reported as 4, 6, or 8, you can assume that the primary and secondary Gleason grades probably are the same. It is rare for a man to have two Gleason grades that are two numbers apart such as $1 + 3$, $2 + 4$, or $3 + 5$.

Extent of cancer found in prostate at surgery: This includes the clinical stage and the status of the tumor margin and prostate capsule.

Clinical stage: As also explained in Chapter 6, the clinical stage is based on what the doctor feels during a DRE. The pathological stage is what is found on the biopsy report. If you do not know it, ask your doctor to provide it to you. The possibilities include T1a, T1b, T1c, T2a, T2b, T2c, T3a, T3b, T4a, and T4b.

Tumor margin: After the prostate is removed, the pathologist will coat the outside of the prostate with ink before processing the tissue. A positive margin means cancer cells are touching the ink.

Extra capsular extension: The capsule is a very thin layer of tissue that surrounds the prostate. Extra capsular extension or penetration means cancer cells are growing outside the capsule.

Seminal vesicle invasion: The seminal vesicles are two small glands attached to the prostate. Seminal vesicle invasion means cancer cells have grown in one or both of seminal vesicles.

Lymph node invasion: The pathology report will state whether lymph nodes were removed during surgery and whether any of them contain cancer. If the lymph nodes were not removed, then leave the box empty.

The Kattan nomogram was developed using results from thousands of patients. It has been rechecked on many other patients and appears to be very reliable. You should realize what it does and does not do. It *does* tell you what happened to a group of men with similar types of tumors as yours. It *does not* tell exactly what will happen to you.

Two cases are shown to illustrate the information provided by this tool. The first patient is 62 years old, his Gleason score is 3 + 3 = 6, the tumor stage is T1c, the tumor margins are negative, the capsule is not penetrated, and the seminal vesicles and lymph nodes do not show cancer. The second patient has a more aggressive cancer. He is 55 years old, his Gleason score is 4 + 4 = 8, the tumor stage is T2b, the tumor margin is positive, and cancer has invaded into the seminal vesicles and the lymph nodes. Both men had their surgery in the last six months.

Examples Using the Kattan Nomogram

Patient Characteristic	Patient 1	Patient 2
Age at surgery	55	62
PSA before surgery (ng/mL)	6	11
Primary Gleason grade	3	4
Secondary Gleason grade	3	4

Examples Using the Kattan Nomogram (Continued)

Patient Characteristic	Patient 1	Patient 2
Clinical stage	T1c	T2b
Tumor margins positive	No	Yes
Extracapsular extension	No	Yes
Cancer in seminal vesicles	No	Yes
Cancer in lymph nodes	No	Yes
Chance of PSA rising above 0.4 ng/mL in 5 years	3%	82%
Chance of PSA rising above 0.4 ng/mL in 10 years	5%	95%
Chance of dying from prostate cancer in 10 years	1%	1%
Chance of dying from prostate cancer in 15 years	1%	2%

The two men have just a slightly different chance of dying from prostate cancer in the next 15 years, but the second man has a much greater chance that his PSA will go up. The information from the Kattan nomogram can help you with your care. If you have a very low risk of developing a rise in your PSA, monitoring can be done less often, perhaps every one or two years. If the PSA does go up, you may not feel the need to have it treated right away because it has a low chance of harming you. If you have a higher risk of recurrence, you would continue to be tested more often and may want to have additional treatment.

A less helpful tool for predicting the likelihood of developing a significant increase in the PSA is a test called the *ultrasensitive PSA*. It can detect smaller amounts of PSA in a blood sample than the standard test. When the level is very low, the chance of your PSA going up is very low. For example, when the ultrasensitive PSA level is below 0.01 ng/mL, the odds of it rising in the next three years are only 4%, but it is almost 90% when the ultrasensitive PSA is at least 0.04 ng/mL.

This tool is not as useful as the Kattan nomogram for several reasons. First, more time is needed after surgery for the PSA to drop to its lowest level. You can have a standard PSA test done in four to six weeks after surgery, but sometimes a longer time is needed before the ultrasensitive PSA can be used. One study found the ultrasensitive PSA took 8 to 10 months before it dropped below 0.01 ng/mL. The only way to be sure that an ultrasensitive PSA level has "bottomed-out" is by performing additional PSA tests several weeks or months later to see if it remains stable. This may cause you considerable anxiety while waiting for that to occur.

A second and more important problem that applies to both predictor tools is doctors do not know what to do with the information. If your ultrasensitive PSA is higher than 0.01 ng/mL, should you get treated immediately or wait until the PSA is rising? Treating all men with this ultrasensitive PSA result would mean many would get a treatment they would never need. For example, treating 100 men with an ultrasensitive PSA of 0.02 ng/mL means that at least 85 are getting unnecessary treatment.

So, if your prostate has been removed and it is time for a check-up, should you have the standard or the ultrasensitive PSA? Until studies report results with longer follow-up, the standard PSA test is sufficient.

What Should You Do if You Have a High Risk for Recurrence?

If you are uncomfortable with the estimated risk of getting a recurrence of your cancer, what should you do? Should you have radiation therapy to the area where the prostate was located, hormone therapy, or both? Only one good study has been done to answer this question. It assigned men to get radiation within 18 weeks of the prostatectomy or be observed until the disease recurred. According to their pathology report, all of them had cancer growing outside their prostate. With more than half the men followed longer than 12.5 years, the key results are the following:

- Metastatic disease occurred in 54% of the men in the control group compared to only 46% in the group getting immediate radiation. These results mean that radiation therapy must be given to about 12 men to prevent one from getting metastatic disease over the next 12.5 years.

- One half of the men treated with radiation lived slightly more than 15 years compared to slightly more than 13 years in the control group. This means about nine men must be treated to prevent one from dying over the next 12.5 years.

- Five years after surgery, hormone therapy was started in 10% of the radiation group compared to 21% in the control group.

- Complications were more common in men receiving radiation including:

  Bowel irritation (proctitis) or rectal bleeding (3% vs 0%)

  Urethral strictures (18% vs 10%)

  Urinary incontinence (7% vs 3%)

- Two years after radiation, both groups had similar bowel and sexual function, but urinary frequency was more common in the group getting radiation.

This study shows a small but definite benefit from immediate radiation. The trade-off is many men get a treatment that does not help them, and they have slightly worse urinary function. You will have to decide if the benefits are worth the risks. If you have cancer outside the prostate and want to do everything possible to survive your cancer, then have the radiation early rather than wait for the PSA to rise. It is even possible that getting radiation today will give better results than in the study. The reason is a higher dose now can be given without causing more side effects.

What to Do if the Prostate-Specific Antigen Is Detectable After Surgery?

In a small percentage of men, the standard PSA does not drop to the desired level after surgery. The reasons could be:

- *Someone else's blood sample was tested.* Though rare, mistakes can occur and most doctors will confirm the result with a second test.

- *Some prostate tissue was left behind.* Although the goal is always to remove the entire prostate, sometimes the surgeon makes a technical error and leaves some prostate tissue in the body. It will make PSA whether it contains normal cells or cancer cells. The only way to find out if cancer is still present is by following the PSA over time or eventually doing a biopsy. Normal cells will produce a very slow rise in the PSA. No other test can tell why the PSA is abnormal.

- *Cancer cells already had spread outside the prostate before the operation.* The pathology report might provide useful information because most pathologists coat the outer surface of the prostate with colored ink before it is processed. When the specimen is viewed under a microscope, cancer cells may be seen touching the ink. This could mean cancer is still in that area.

- *Cancer has spread to some other area of the body.* They continue producing PSA after the prostate is gone which prevents the PSA from dropping to the desired level. If the PSA continues to rise, either a bone scan or Prostascint scan may eventually show where the cancer is located.

How do you decide what to do if this happens to you? The first thing to know is you are in no immediate danger, but it does mean your PSA is likely to keep going up. Should you have radiation therapy, hormone therapy, or both? In the study discussed earlier in this chapter, about one third of the men had a PSA above 0.2 ng/mL following surgery. Getting radiation within three months also improved their survival. This means radiation also helps men with a measurable PSA after surgery. Good studies have not yet been done to find out if adding hormone therapy to the radiation will make things even better. Even so, it is an option with side effects that may affect your quality-of-life.

Another option is to *not get radiation right away*, but instead wait to see if and when your PSA eventually goes up. It may allow you to avoid getting an unnecessary treatment. At this time, doctors do not know if starting the radiation then will be as helpful as getting it very soon after surgery but good studies are being done.

Studies also are needed before you can be told exactly what to expect by adding hormone therapy. The key thing to remember is radiation helps some men but it does have trade-offs.

The Bottom Line About Radical Prostatectomy

Every treatment you read about in this book has reasons to choose it and reasons to avoid it. Surgery is the right choice if you want the most aggressive treatment for your cancer, providing you are willing to accept the possible side effects. More information is available about the results with surgery than any other option. Every other treatment except brachytherapy has been used for less than 10 years. That means their long-term results are more uncertain. You must realize, however, that no good study has proved that surgery definitely is better than any of the other options. Knowing the right questions to ask is the best thing you can do to decide if surgery is right for you.

Removing the Lymph Nodes: If, When, and How?

If you have decided to have a radical prostatectomy, be aware of another controversy. What should you do about your lymph nodes? Should they be removed or left alone? If cancer has spread into the lymph nodes, which is called *lymph node metastases*, should the prostate still be removed or should it be left in your body and another treatment be given? A debate persists because studies do not provide definite answers.

How can doctors tell if cancer is in your lymph nodes? The only reliable way is to take them out and examine them under a microscope by doing an operation called a *pelvic lymphadenectomy* or *pelvic lymph node dissection* (PLND). A pathologist can check them immediately by doing *frozen sections*, which takes about 15 to 30 minutes, or get the results in one or two days by doing *permanent sections*. Some surgeons will wait for the results of the frozen sections before completing the prostatectomy. If they are *negative*, meaning cancer is not present, then the prostatectomy is completed. If they are *positive*, meaning cancer is in the lymph nodes, the prostate is not removed, the wound is closed, and a different treatment is done after the person recovers from surgery.

Other doctors take a more aggressive approach. They remove the lymph nodes and the prostate without doing frozen sections.

This decision is based on one study of men with cancer in their lymph nodes. The results *suggested* that taking out the prostate and giving immediate hormone therapy might help some men live longer than delaying that treatment. Another reason to do both operations is that even if a man does not live longer, removing the prostate would reduce his risk of developing urinary obstruction in the future.

This debate has changed considerably since the discovery of the prostate-specific antigen (PSA) test. So far, doctors have no proof that men benefit from having normal lymph nodes removed. Now, very few men have cancer in their lymph nodes when their cancer is detected so doctors can be more selective and avoid putting many men through an unnecessary operation. They will do a pelvic lymphadenectomy only if the odds are high that the cancer has spread into the lymph nodes.

There is another good argument against doing a pelvic lymphadenectomy in everyone. Prostate cancer does not always spread in an orderly fashion. Sometimes it spreads into the lymph nodes very close to the prostate and in other cases, it skips those areas and invades further away.

Lymph nodes are named according to a nearby blood vessel. Those closest to the prostate are called the *external iliac and obturator* nodes, followed by the *hypogastric, internal iliac, and presacral nodes,* and then the *common iliac and aortic nodes.* In the past, only the external iliac and obturator nodes were removed. The operation is called a *limited pelvic lymphadenectomy.* Doctors thought that if the lymph nodes near the prostate were negative, then the others also would not contain cancer.

Recent studies changed this thinking. They showed that prostate cancer sometimes skips the lymph nodes near the prostate and invades others further away. That means some men will be diagnosed incorrectly if only the limited operation is done. Those men might get the wrong treatment. Checking all the lymph nodes requires doing an *extended pelvic lymphadenectomy.*

The only problem is, it has several disadvantages including the following:

- It takes longer to perform.

- The pathologist needs more time to do the frozen sections, making the entire operation take longer.

- The complication rate is slightly higher compared to the limited operation.

What Are the Complications of a Pelvic Lymph Node Dissection?

Although the complication rate of removing the lymph nodes is much lower today than it was 20 years ago, some that occur still are very serious. Of course, the frequency of side effects will vary depending on the surgeon. The results from one good study of men having a limited dissection are shown in the next table.

Complications of PLND	Frequency
Injury to bowel	1%
Injury to obturator nerve	1%–2%
Deep venous thrombosis	5%–6%
Lymphocele	9%–11%
Pulmonary embolism	1%–2%

Some of these complications could be due to taking out the prostate along with the lymph nodes because both were done at the same time. Very little information is available about the frequency of side effects in men having a PLND without the prostatectomy.

Injuries to the bowel and obturator nerve are not serious, providing they are recognized and repaired at the time of surgery. However, the other three complications can be serious. A *lymphocele* is a collection of fluid where the lymph nodes were removed occurring several days after the prostate is removed. It can get infected and cause pain. It is treated by inserting a needle to drain the fluid. A *deep venous thrombosis* or *DVT* is a blood clot that forms in the leg, resulting in swelling and pain. It requires a short hospitalization and blood thinners for six months. Sometimes it leads to a blood clot in the lung called a *pulmonary embolism*, which can be life threatening.

Should You Have the Lymph Nodes Removed?

Doctors have their own opinion about what to do about the lymph nodes. But to get the treatment that is right for you, the decision should be shared with your doctor. To do that, you need to know your odds or chances of having lymph node metastases.

Two tools have been developed for this purpose, but do not expect your doctor to use either of them. Most of them will simply estimate your odds. One popular tool is called the *Partin tables*, which can be found for free on the Web by typing those words into your browser. It can provide the following information about your cancer:

- The odds it is confined inside the prostate.

- The odds it has grown outside the prostate.

- The odds it has invaded into the seminal vesicles.

- The odds it has spread to the lymph nodes.

Some example results are shown in the following table:

Partin Table Results

PSA	Clinical Stage	Gleason Score	Probability of Lymph Node Metastases
0–10 ng/mL	T1C, T2a	5 or 6	0%–1%
0–10 ng/mL	T1C	3 + 4 = 7	1%–3%
More than 10 ng/mL	T1C	4 + 3 = 7	5%–17%
More than 10 ng/mL	T2a	8–10	5%–22%

When you arrive at the Web site, select "Partin Tables" on the right side of the screen. You then enter your PSA, the clinical stage of your tumor, and the Gleason score from the biopsy. Select "calculate" and it will immediately tell you your results.

Another popular option for calculating the chance of having lymph node metastases is the *Kattan Nomogram* (www.mskcc.org). Begin by selecting "prostate cancer" from the drop-down menu for "type of cancer," click on "prostate cancer prediction tool," then on "open calculator." Lastly, select "Pretreatment." Under "Primary Treatment Outcome" select "Progression-free Probability After Radical Prostatectomy." You then will be asked to enter your age, PSA, primary and secondary Gleason grade or your Gleason score, and the number of biopsy needles showing cancer and not showing cancer. You can ask your doctor for a copy of your biopsy report to get some of this information. After everything is entered, hit "Calculate" and it will show you the chance of having lymph node metastases.

Both the Partin and Kattan calculators are very accurate for men with a Gleason score between 2 and 6; they slightly underestimate the risk for a Gleason score of 7 and greatly underestimate it for Gleason score of 8 to 10.

Fortunately, more than 80% of all new cases diagnosed today have only a 0% to 1% chance of cancer in the lymph nodes. If these are your odds, removing the lymph nodes makes *no sense.* Your chance of having an unnecessary operation is 99%. The only good reason to remove the lymph nodes is if the doctor feels something suspicious at the time of the surgery.

Even when your odds of benefitting are this low, do not be surprised if your doctor still plans to remove some of them. Be aware that the only person benefitting is the surgeon because more money will be collected from you and your insurance company. Removing normal lymph nodes will not improve your survival.

If you do ask your doctor what is planned and are told that some lymph nodes will be removed, you should ask, "Can you please explain how I will benefit given my small chance of having metastases?" If your odds of lymph node metastases are very low, you can request they be left alone.

Suppose your odds of having lymph node metastases are not very low, what should you do? One study suggested that the potential benefits of a PLND outweigh the potential risks when the chance of lymph node metastases is at least 15%. This is not a hard-and-fast rule, and there is no definite right or wrong answer. If you do decide to have a PLND, your next question should be, "Will you do a limited or extended PLND?" Remember, an extended PLND will be needed to get the most accurate result. If you are not satisfied with the answers to these questions, then you might consider getting a second opinion.

What to Do if Cancer Is in the Lymph Nodes?

Doctors continue to disagree about the best treatment for men with lymph node metastases. The options depend on whether they are found on the frozen sections or several days after the prostate is removed. When metastases are found on the frozen sections, the options include the following:

- Leave the prostate in place and give immediate or delayed hormone therapy.

- Take out the prostate and give hormone therapy immediately or after the cancer progresses.

- Leave the prostate in place and give radiation combined with immediate or delayed hormone therapy.

Because no well-done studies have been done, all the options are reasonable. If you want to be conservative, then leave the prostate in place and delay the hormone treatment, but if you want to be aggressive, then take out the prostate and start hormone therapy right away.

If the lymph node metastases are discovered several days after the prostate is removed, then your choices are immediate or delayed hormone therapy. Although many studies have been published, only one was randomized. It has been criticized because it did not enroll as many men as planned, which may have biased the results. At 10 years, men getting immediate hormone therapy had a significantly better survival compared to those who delayed getting the hormone treatment.

Because the study was done before the discovery of the PSA test, doctors do not know if hormone therapy still must be started right away or the same benefit would occur by starting it when the PSA level starts to rise. The bottom line here is all these options also are reasonable, but if you want to be more aggressive with your treatment, then start the hormone treatment right away.

The Bottom Line

You should be a part of the decision about your lymph nodes. If you want to do everything possible that might improve your survival, then have the lymph nodes and the prostate removed. Do not bother having frozen sections done, but you should have an extended pelvic lymphadenectomy.

If instead you want a more balanced approach that avoids unnecessary risk, then be more selective. Do not have the lymph nodes removed unless your odds of lymph node metastases are at least 10%. If they are removed, then it should be done by an extended PLND with frozen sections. Your prostate should be removed only if the lymph nodes are negative. Here again, the best advice is to discuss this with your surgeon and ask the necessary questions.

External Beam Radiation

Several terms are used to describe radiation therapy including *external beam radiation, radiotherapy, XRT, and EBRT.* This treatment has gone through many changes over the past 20 years resulting in more options with fewer complications. The challenge is trying to decide which approach is a good option for treating localized prostate cancer. The reason for the difficulty is that well-designed studies comparing external radiation to other treatments have never been done. Also, the methods and amount of radiation used has been changing. That means you will have to learn about the strengths and weaknesses of this approach so you can decide if radiation is right for you.

What Is Radiation and How Does It Work?

Before discussing the details of the different types of radiation available, you should know some basics about what it is and how it works. Radiation is a type of energy. It can occur naturally like the radiation from the sun or it can be man-made like the energy from your microwave oven. The sun's energy comes from *waves,* and the energy from *uranium* used in nuclear power plants comes from very fast-moving tiny *particles.* The level or intensity of the energy determines how it affects our body. For example, a microwave produces a low level of wave energy making it very safe. In contrast, the sun produces very high-energy waves, making it potentially more dangerous.

External beam radiation is a treatment that uses a machine to deliver rays of high energy. It works on the *DNA*, which is contained in all living cells. DNA controls the ability of cells to divide. Cancer cells harm us because they continue to divide without stopping. The energy from radiation machines is so strong that it can damage the DNA in cancer cells, causing them to die or making them unable to divide.

The tiny particles that deliver energy differ in their ability to penetrate our skin. Some do not penetrate at all whereas other particles easily pass through the body. Radiation that passes deeper through the skin is better for treating cancers inside our body. Cancers are treated with *alpha, beta,* and *neutron* particles, and *gamma* and *x-ray* waves. Prostate cancer is most commonly treated using gamma rays.

What Are the Benefits and Risks of External Radiation?

The advantage of external radiation is it may cure your disease without having an operation. The potential disadvantages include the side effects that may occur, the chance that some cancer cells will survive, and the difficulty of doing surgery if the cancer is not eliminated. Also, some studies suggest that radiation slightly increases the risk of developing bladder or rectal cancer more than 5 or 10 years after the treatment. It might affect one or two men out of every 1,000 receiving radiation. At this time, doctors do not know if the newer methods of delivering radiation will have the same risk. The most common side effects of radiation are shown in the following table.

Side Effects of External Radiation
Impotence
Incontinence
Bowel dysfunction (diarrhea, bloody stool, urgency)

Side Effects of External Radiation (Continued)

Sexual dysfunction

Hematuria

Bowel changes may begin within a few weeks of starting treatment and gradually go away in several months in most men. A small percentage continue to have problems permanently. Sexual dysfunction, incontinence, and hematuria may not fully develop until one or two years later. Some uncontrolled studies tried to compare the frequency of these side effects in men treated by surgery, radical prostatectomy, and seed implantation. Doctors often use these studies to support one treatment over another. The results are not shown here because the groups are not very similar meaning the treatments cannot be accurately compared. Some of the differences between men getting each treatment include the following:

- age

- general health

- sexual and urinary function

- dose of radiation

- physician's experience

Making conclusions is nearly impossible when studies include men that differ in so many ways. Rather than quote you percentages that may be inaccurate, your best course of action is to ask the doctor for the results seen in his or her patients. Remember to ask how they got the results. Written surveys filled out by patients are much more accurate than asking patients questions when they are in the office.

Options for External Radiation

Many options are available for treating men with external radiation. The list includes the following:

- external beam radiation therapy (EBRT)

- 3-dimensional conformal radiation therapy (3D-CRT)

- intensity-modulated radiation therapy (IMRT)

- proton beam therapy (PBT)

- the CyberKnife robotic system

- IMRT using the Calypso tracking system

External Beam Radiation Therapy

Of all the options, this one has been used for the longest time. Before treatment can begin, a computerized axial tomography (CAT) scan is done so the radiation therapist can create a treatment plan. The size and shape of your prostate will determine where the radiation will be given and how much will be used. Radiation is measured in units called a *rad* or *gray*. Rad stands for *radiation absorbed dose* and gray is a metric term abbreviated as Gy that is being used more often for prostate cancer. A body mold will be made of your pelvic and reused to keep you in the same position for each treatment.

Traditional external beam is delivered by a *linear accelerator* or *LINAC*. The radiation is aimed at the prostate and extends a few millimeters beyond the outer capsule to help ensure that all the cancer cells are killed. Each day you will lie on a table and then an x-ray is taken to make sure you are in the proper position. Treatment is given once a day, five days a week until the total amount is delivered, which takes about six weeks. Each treatment is completed in about 15 minutes and afterward you can resume all your activities.

The total dose delivered with EBRT is from 66 to 70 Gy, usually from four directions around your body. The beams are delivered in the shape of a square or rectangle. Because the prostate has neither of those shapes, normal tissues often receive some radiation, which increases the chance of getting side effects. Traditional EBRT at those doses is now rarely used to treat this disease because studies showed that it often failed to kill all the cancer cells. Higher doses cannot be given because it causes too many side effects.

3-Dimensional Conformal Radiation Therapy

Improvements in the LINAC equipment have made it possible to focus the radiation beams more directly on the prostate and less on the surrounding tissues. Patients benefit by being able to receive a higher dose of radiation to the tumor with fewer complications. 3D-CRT is done using computers, which plan the treatment from different angles to the body according to the shape of the prostate. The dose used with this approach ranges from about 68 to 81 Gy.

Intensity-Modulated Radiation Therapy

The next improvement was a modification of 3D-CRT. The radiation is broken up into a large number of narrow beams rather than a single wide beam. The intensity of radiation with each beam is adjustable, allowing greater control of the dose given to the prostate and the surrounding organs. The net result of IMRT is more radiation reaches the cancer without greatly increasing the amount hitting the bladder or rectum. A CAT scan is performed to plan the treatment and a body mold is made to keep you in the same position while you are treated.

CyberKnife Robotic System

Another new development has been the use of a robotic instrument to deliver IMRT from almost any angle to the body. With standard IMRT, the treatment is planned based on a single CAT scan done before the treatment begins. Each day, however, the prostate may be in a slightly different position due to the bladder filling with urine or the rectum filling with air and stool. This can result in *undertreating* the cancer or *overtreating* the surrounding tissues. The entire treatment takes many days to complete because the daily dose must be limited. Otherwise, too many side effects will occur.

The CyberKnife robot works differently. It takes multiple images during treatment and then a computer adjusts each thin beam of radiation to hit the intended target. The exact position of the prostate is identified using several markers placed inside the gland about one week before the treatment is started. They are inserted under ultrasound guidance. The benefits of this approach are more radiation can be given each day and the entire treatment can be completed in about one week. Each treatment takes about 35 to 45 minutes. It sounds like a very good approach to treat prostate cancer but so far, little information is available about long-term survival or complications.

The Calypso Tracking System

In 2006, a machine became available that was designed to improve IMRT radiation by adjusting for any movement of the prostate. It is similar to the CyberKnife system in having tiny sensors placed inside the gland before the treatment begins. These sensors send off signals 10 times per second that deliver information about the location of the prostate. It functions like a Global Positioning System (GPS) that you may use in the car to guide you to a destination. Some call this a "GPS for the body."

The Calypso tracking system alerts the physician if the prostate moves by more than a few millimeters. When that happens, the treatment is stopped allowing time to reposition the radiation beam. The Calypso system permits higher doses of radiation to be given. The expectation is that side effects will not increase but since this machine only received approval in 2006, long-term results will not be ready for some time.

Proton Beam Radiation

This type of radiation generates energy using *protons* from a proton accelerator instead of gamma rays from a LINAC. The difference is that radiation from a LINAC delivers its energy as it passes *through* the tissues. That means normal tissue is getting some of the energy. Protons only deliver their energy when they *reach* the target. The result is proton beam radiation *may* deliver less radiation outside the prostate. The theoretical but as yet unproven advantage of PBT is that it may cause fewer side effects. Potentially, more radiation could be given to the tumor. Ten-year survival rates have not yet been reported.

Which Type of Radiation Should You Receive?

With so many options for getting radiation for your prostate cancer, you now want to know, "Which method is best?" The answer is not available right now because no good studies have compared them. Also, few of them have long-term results available. Because prostate cancer often grows slowly, these treatments cannot be compared unless the patients have been followed for many years. Valid conclusions cannot be made based on short-term results. Even though they are not available, you still can get some guidance on what to do.

First, if you decide that radiation is for you, make sure that newer equipment is being used. The older LINAC machines are no longer adequate. After reading about the differences between 3D-CRT and IMRT, you might want to know, "Is IMRT better?" Uncontrolled studies *suggest* a slightly lower percentage of bowel side effects with IMRT but no difference in urinary side effects. Without good evidence that IMRT is definitely better, either approach is reasonable. Still, if both are available and you have a choice, IMRT *might* give you a better result.

What about CyberKnife, IMRT using the Calypso tracking system, and PBT? They all have theoretical advantages over 3D-CRT and IMRT but not one comparison has been done and no long-term survival results have been reported. The Calypso tracking system should be as effective as IMRT, but it is too early to tell if it is safer or delivers better results.

Despite the lack of long-term results, hospitals and doctors are heavily marketing the newer methods. These promotions make you believe that they are as good as or better than IMRT or 3D-CRT. The truth is no one knows. Despite this uncertainty, getting treated using one of them is not necessarily a bad choice for you but it does mean you really do not know what to expect from them. They may give very good results, but they also could prove to be inferior or cause more side effects. Hopefully, information will become available soon.

Until that time, the following comments may be helpful for deciding what to do. Proton beam radiation has the longest track record of these newer options. It has been used to treat thousands of patients over the last 15 years. Despite this experience, only one study has been published. It reported PSA results at seven years but it did not report survival results nor assess side effects using written surveys. Therefore, proton beam could be as good, better, or worse than IMRT but there is no way to know. It is more costly, and it is not available in every city because of the cost of building the machines, although more are becoming available. You may have to travel if you want it done. At this time, there is no evidence that it is a better approach than the other options.

The CyberKnife robotic system offers the greatest advantage over the newer options because it can be completed very quickly. The entire treatment takes only one week. You may find that very appealing and worth trying, but you should understand that its long-term effects are unknown.

Your choice of radiation methods should depend on your goals and motivation. If you are willing to try something new without knowing exactly how well it works, then any of these options can be selected. If you want a more established treatment, then 3D-CRT or IMRT would be a better choice right now.

Regardless of the type you choose, information is accumulating about how much radiation you should get. One well-done study assigned men with localized prostate cancer to receive either 70.2 Gy or 79.2 Gy. With more than one half of them followed for about nine years, the survival rates are about the same. One difference is fewer men with a low-risk cancer had a rise in their prostate-specific antigen (PSA) level if they got the higher dose.

Another good study compared men's quality-of-life three years after getting 68 Gy or 78 Gy and found no difference. Does that mean you are better off getting a higher dose of radiation? At this time, the answer is not clear. The PSA is not a reliable way to predict long-term survival results. Still, most doctors are recommending a dose greater than 72 Gy because it can be done very safely. For now, a higher dose of radiation may do a better job of getting rid of your cancer. Doctors still don't know if it will cause more long-term side effects or help you live longer. If you decide to have radiation, be sure to ask the doctor how much they plan to give you in addition to what equipment they use. If your goal is to avoid any problems from prostate cancer, then a higher dose may be best without making your quality-of-life worse.

Treating Low-, Intermediate-, and High-Risk Prostate Cancer With Radiation

One way doctors are trying to compare different treatments is to separate tumors into groups based on their ability to spread. Low-risk prostate cancers are those with a PSA level less than 10 ng/mL, a digital rectal exam (DRE) showing T1 or T2a disease (see Chapter 6), and a Gleason score less than 7. The good news is any of the methods for giving external radiation may be considered because these tumors do not pose much risk over the next 10 to 15 years.

The best candidates are men with a life expectancy of more than 10 years who want to maximize their survival. Many doctors now are concerned that low-risk cancers are being overtreated.

Until they can predict which ones are dangerous, you will have to decide if the benefits of radiation outweigh its risks. The safest approach is to have IMRT or 3D-CRT rather than EBRT. What about the dose of radiation? As explained previously, 70 Gy is not enough, but the best dose has not been determined. Most doctors will use a higher dose to treat a low-risk tumor.

Intermediate risk cancers have one of the following characteristics:

- PSA level between 10 and 20 ng/mL

- stage T2b

- Gleason score = 7

Two good studies have tested whether combining hormone therapy with radiation would be better than radiation alone. One study used two months of hormone therapy before, two months during, and two months after radiation for a total of six months. Most of the men had intermediate risk tumors. At five years, the overall survival was about 10% higher in those getting radiation combined with hormone therapy.

A second study tested two months of hormone therapy before and during radiation in men with intermediate risk tumors and found a significant benefit. The estimated survival rate at eight years was 72% in men getting both radiation and hormones, but only 66% in men getting radiation alone. That means for every 100 men who get hormone therapy with their radiation, six are prevented from dying.

At the time this study was done, 66 to 70 Gy was being used to treat localized prostate cancer. Many doctors have asked whether the hormone therapy was helpful because the dose of radiation was too low. Now that a higher dose of radiation has become the standard, perhaps the hormone therapy is not necessary. Without doing another study, however, doctors cannot be sure.

For now, if you want to have the best chance of surviving your intermediate risk cancer, then it makes sense for you to get between four and six months of hormone therapy even if you get more than

70 Gy of radiation. The hormone therapy consists of two drugs. One is an injection called a *luteinizing hormone-releasing hormone* (LHRH) *agonist*, which works by lowering testosterone. The other is a pill called an *antiandrogen*, which stops testosterone from stimulating cancer cells. They are described in detail in Chapters 25 and 26. Good studies suggest that higher doses reduce the chance that the PSA level will go up, but it also increases the odds of having bowel side effects.

High-risk localized prostate cancers include men with a Gleason score of 8, 9, or 10 or a PSA level of more than 20 ng/mL, or stage T2c. These tumors are more difficult to treat. Radiation often is not successful because almost 80% of these tumors are growing outside the prostate. Many doctors believe one therapy alone is not enough to treat a high-risk cancer.

Several well-done studies tested a combination of hormone therapy and 70 Gy of radiation in men with "harder to treat" disease. It significantly improved survival compared to radiation alone or hormone therapy alone. In the best study done so far, survival was 18% higher in men receiving hormone therapy for three years starting when radiation began. About 10% of them had high-risk localized cancer and the remainder were thought to have cancer growing outside the prostate gland. Another study is needed to confirm that men with high-risk localized disease really benefit from this approach.

Another well-done study found that men with a Gleason 8, 9, or 10 cancer had a much better survival if they received radiation and 28 months of hormone therapy compared to only four months. The hormone therapy consisted of the LHRH agonist by itself or combined with one month of an antiandrogen.

As expected, the addition of hormone therapy increased the rate of side effects including hot flashes, a decreased sex drive, and decreased sexual function. These side effects decrease after the hormone therapy is stopped but they do not always disappear.

What should you do if you have high-risk localized prostate cancer? Again, if your goal is to have the best chance of surviving your cancer, then get hormone therapy for 28 to 36 months along with your radiation. Drugs are available to help you if the hormone therapy causes side effects.

Some doctors argue that the only reason hormone therapy was helpful in these studies is because the dose of radiation was too low. For that reason, they believe you should not take hormone therapy when you get more than 70 Gy of radiation. Others will say that the combination is clearly good for men with cancer outside the prostate, but there is not enough proof that it helps men with high-risk localized disease. Perhaps one day, a perfect study will be done. Until then, the best information available provides very good support for getting hormone therapy together with radiation for a high-risk cancer.

Some doctors have used a combination of external radiation and brachytherapy to treat localized prostate cancer, even adding hormone therapy. Little information is available to assess how often side effects occur or whether it is better than a combination of external radiation and hormone therapy. Therefore, it cannot be recommended as a better treatment option at this time.

Monitoring Patients After Radiation

The PSA test is the best test for monitoring patients treated with any form of radiation therapy. Most doctors measure the PSA level beginning three months after completion of the radiation. How often should it be done? Doctors tend to individualize their practice because no studies show any particular approach is better. A reasonable approach is to measure the PSA level every three months for one or two years and then decrease it to every six months. Beyond five years, it can be done once a year unless it is increasing. Most doctors also do a DRE to determine if the cancer is growing. That probably is unnecessary because the PSA test is more reliable. If the DRE feels abnormal but the PSA is not increasing, then you are highly unlikely to have recurrent cancer. A bone scan and CAT scan is not done until the PSA level exceeds 10 ng/mL. The only reason to have a bone scan sooner is if you develop bone pain.

One difference between surgery and radiation is the PSA level declines more slowly after radiation. It may not reach its lowest level, called the nadir, for up to two years after treatment has been completed. Some men feel very anxious when the PSA level does not drop right away. Knowing that the decline takes time should make you a little more comfortable. Some patients ask if a slowly dropping PSA level predicts a worse result. Currently, there is no good evidence that the rate of decline in the PSA level has any impact on the cancer coming back.

Researchers are working on ways to predict what will happen after radiation the same way predictions are made after surgery. Several problems may complicate this task. Most importantly, the radiation used in the past has changed. That means what happened to those patients may not predict what will happen to patients treated by current methods. The changes include increasing doses of radiation, the selective use of hormone therapy, and different ways to administer the radiation such as 3D-CRT and IMRT.

Some predictions are possible using the nadir PSA. Not all men get the same nadir PSA. Usually, lower is better. One study separated men into two groups based on their PSA level two years after completing radiation. The results are shown in the following table.

Chance of Developing Metastatic Disease Following External Beam Radiation

PSA Result Two Years After Radiation	Metastases at Five Years	Metastases at 10 Years
0–1.5 ng/mL	2.4%	7.9%
More than 1.5 ng/mL	10%	17.9%

Men with a PSA level less than 1.5 ng/mL at two years had much better results. They were much less likely to get widespread cancer at 5 and 10 years after radiation. This was a retrospective study so it is not as reliable as a randomized study. Still, it should provide some comfort to you if your PSA level stays low.

The Bottom Line About External Radiation

External radiation is a reasonable option to treat your localized prostate cancer if you have at least a 10-year life expectancy and you wish to avoid surgery. One difference compared to surgery is well-done studies have shown that hormone therapy combined with radiation improves survival in intermediate and high-risk prostate cancer. Recently, a large review was conducted of medical studies published in the last few years. The goal was to find out the results of well done randomized studies. Two major conclusions resulted from this study.

1. No study has proven that any form of radiation resulted in better survival compared to watchful waiting in men with localized disease.

2. No study has been done to determine whether one form of radiation is superior to any of the other radiation methods.

At this time, no conclusion can be made about whether radiation is better, worse, or the same as radical prostatectomy. Like all the other options, this treatment has pros and cons. Radical prostatectomy may be a better choice if you are young, very healthy, and have a life expectancy of at least 15 years and hope to do everything possible to avoid dying from prostate cancer. The reason is long-term results with the latest radiation equipment are not yet available.

Brachytherapy

Another way to deliver radiation to the prostate is called brachytherapy. In Latin, the word *brachy* means short distance, which is appropriate for a treatment in which the radioactive material is placed very close to the cancer. It works like external radiation by damaging cancer cells so they die or become unable to divide.

This treatment can be done in two ways. One option is to leave the source of radiation in the body, which is called *permanent brachytherapy*. The other option is to place it in the prostate for a short time and then remove it, which is called *temporary brachytherapy*. The radioactive materials used for permanent brachytherapy are *iodine 125* (^{125}I), *palladium 103* (^{103}Pd), and *cesium 131* (^{131}Cs) whereas temporary brachytherapy is done using *iridium 192* (^{192}Ir).

One of the differences between these materials is how long the radiation will last. The *half-life* is the number of days it takes for 50% of the radiation to disappear. For ^{125}I, it is 60 days, ^{103}Pd is next at 17 days, and it is only 9.7 days for ^{131}Cs. This means ^{125}I loses about 97% of its radiation in 300 days compared to 85 days for ^{103}Pd and 49 days for ^{131}Cs.

Another way that these materials differ is the intensity or strength of radiation they deliver to the body. This is measured as the *dose rate*. A low dose rate or LDR means the material gives off small amounts of radiation each day. A high dose rate or HDR means a large amount is given off. ^{125}I, ^{103}Pd, and ^{131}Cs have LDRs, which is the reason they can be put in the body permanently. ^{192}Ir has a much higher dose rate so it can only be put in the body for a short time.

Permanent Brachytherapy

The radioactive material used for permanent brachytherapy is contained inside tiny "seeds" or tubes made of titanium. They look like birdseeds, each one measuring a few millimeters in length. That is why the treatment is often called *seed implantation*. Prostate brachytherapy began in the 1970s, but it was not very successful because the seeds were placed by hand during an open operation. The development of transrectal ultrasound in the 1980s significantly improved the technique because the seeds could be placed more accurately and without having to perform an open operation.

What Are the Advantages and Disadvantages of Permanent Brachytherapy?

The main advantage of permanent brachytherapy compared to external radiation is a higher dose of radiation can be given to the prostate. The total dose is about 145 Gy for ^{125}I, 125 Gy for ^{103}Pd, and 115 Gy for ^{131}Cs. Other advantages are that it is completed quickly, causes few side effects during the first few months after treatment, and it allows you to resume all your activities in just a few days. The disadvantages are the potential short-term and long-term side effects that may occur and the possibility that the cancer may not be completely destroyed. Also, removing the prostate is more difficult should the tumor recur.

Side Effects of Permanent Brachytherapy
Urinary retention
Urinary incontinence
Urinary frequency
Blood in urine
Erectile dysfunction
Bowel dysfunction
Urethral stricture
Seed migration to the lung or bladder

Side effects after permanent brachytherapy depend on many factors including the following:

- the experience of the doctor doing it
- your age and health
- the radiation material used for the implant

The most common short-term side effects are urinary frequency, urgency, difficulty emptying the bladder, and blood in the stool. They occur within the first few weeks after the implant and gradually improve. Blood in the stool usually resolves without any treatment. Some men also complain of a dry orgasm meaning that no fluid comes out.

The chances of having urinary problems after treatment partly depend on your urinary function before treatment. A questionnaire called the International Prostate Symptom Score or IPSS is used to measure urinary symptoms (see the following table). It has seven questions, each with five possible answers so the score can range from 0 to 35. You can do the survey and find out your score.

IPSS Questionnaire

	Not at all (0)	Less than 1 in 5 (1)	Less than half the time (2)	About half the time (3)	More than half the time (4)	Almost always (5)
Over the past month, how often have you had a sensation of not emptying your bladder completely after you finish urinating?						
Over the past month, how often have you had to urinate again less than two hours after urinating?						
Over the past month, how often have you found you stopped and started again several times when you urinate?						
Over the past month, how often have you found it difficult to postpone urination?						
Over the past month, how often have you had a weak urinary stream?						

IPSS Questionnaire (Continued)

	Not at all (0)	Less than 1 in 5 (1)	Less than half the time (2)	About half the time (3)	More than half the time (4)	Almost always (5)
Over the past month, how often have you had to push or strain to begin urination?						
Over the past month, how many times did you most typically get up to urinate from the time you went to bed at night until you got up in the morning?	0 /night	1 /night	2 /night	3 /night	4 /night	5 or more /night
Total Score						

A higher IPSS score means you are having more urinary symptoms. Doctors have learned that the urinary complications after brachytherapy are much higher in men that have an IPSS score of more than 15 before treatment.

The urinary symptoms resulting from brachytherapy are caused by inflammation in the urethra. Occasionally this leads to a complete blockage called urinary retention. The blockage is relieved by passing a rubber tube called a urethral catheter into the penis. The tube is connected to a bag that collects the urine, which you empty when it is full. The inflammation usually goes away within a few weeks, and the catheter can be removed. In some cases, anti-inflammatory drugs such as steroids are prescribed.

Brachytherapy can have long-term effects on your bladder, bowel, and sexual function. They can develop soon after treatment and persist, or occasionally they develop up to one to two years later. If bloody stool persists, a biopsy of the rectal wall should be avoided because it can result in a *fistula*, which is an opening in the rectum that allows bowel contents to leak out.

The frequency of side effects is most accurately determined using written surveys, but most doctors do not use them. If you are considering this treatment, make sure to ask about the results obtained by your doctor and whether surveys were used. Some survey results are presented in Chapter 18.

What Are the Results Following Permanent Brachytherapy?

No doubt you want to know how prostate brachytherapy compares with other treatments. If you have already read about some of the other treatments described in other chapters, you should not be surprised to find out that this treatment also has never been compared in a properly done study. As an alternative you might ask, "What percentage of men are alive 10 years after having brachytherapy?" Even that question is nearly impossible to answer because few doctors have reported long-term results. They have only been *estimated*, which is much less reliable.

As mentioned in previous chapters, the best way to compare treatments is to separate cancers into low-, intermediate-, and high-risk groups. This is done based on the prostate-specific antigen (PSA) level, the Gleason score, and the clinical stage. The most commonly used definitions for localized disease are the following:

- **Low-risk disease**—Patients have a PSA level less than 10 ng/mL, a Gleason score less than 7 and a clinical stage of T1 or T2a.

- **Intermediate-risk disease**—Patients have a PSA level of greater than 10 ng/mL, a Gleason score of 7, or a clinical stage of T2b.

- **High-risk disease**—Patients have a PSA level over 20 ng/ml, a Gleason score of 8, 9, or 10 or a clinical stage of T2c.

Sadly, few studies separate patients into these groups when reporting long-term results, which is another reason why comparing this
treatment to others is difficult.

The most important result from a treatment is the survival rate,
which is the percentage of men who are alive years after the treatment. Because prostate cancer usually grows slowly, at least 10-year
survival rates are needed to compare different treatments. Because
most men haven't been followed that long, doctors instead report
the percentage of men that didn't get a rise in their PSA level. This
is called the *biochemical disease-free survival* (BDFS). This is not nearly as
helpful as survival results because of the following:

- Many men also were given hormone therapy or external
  radiation, which can make the PSA results look better.

- The definition used for a rising PSA level is not a reliable way
  to predict what will happen to survival.

- Most studies estimate the results using statistical methods,
  which can give misleading information. The reason is many
  men have not been followed very long.

You should realize that estimating PSA results at 10 years in low-
risk cancers is not very helpful because similar results are seen in
men who don't get any treatment. The bottom line is that no reliable conclusion can be made about the long-term survival after
brachytherapy. It could be as good, better than, or worse than other
treatments. Without a proper study, you should know that most
doctors believe *this treatment is as reasonable an option as radical prostatectomy
and external radiation, particularly for men with low-risk disease.*

What about doing permanent brachytherapy for intermediate-
or high-risk cancers? Often, these groups are treated with a combination of brachytherapy and external radiation and/or hormone
therapy. The problem again is 15-year survival results are not available. Also, no good studies show that these combinations are definitely better than either one alone. Studies are underway to get this

information. Until then, the value of combining these treatments for men with intermediate or high-risk cancer could be as good, better, or inferior to other options. Doctors cannot be sure what to tell you at this time.

Who Is a Good Candidate for Permanent Brachytherapy?

Although brachytherapy by itself is a reasonable option for men with localized prostate cancer, it is not for everyone. The most important requirements are that you are healthy enough to be able to have general anesthesia and your life expectancy should be at least 10 years. Brachytherapy might not be an ideal choice if your life expectancy is more than 15 years and your goal is to live as long as possible. The reason is little is known about the percentage of men surviving for that number of years. That means the treatment has more uncertainty than radical prostatectomy.

Prostate size is a very important requirement for permanent brachytherapy. Some doctors set an upper limit of only 40 cc (cubic centimeters) whereas others will treat a prostate up to 60 cc. If your prostate is above these limits, you still may be a candidate if *hormone therapy* drugs can shrink the gland to the required size. These drugs lower your testosterone level and can decrease the prostate size by about 30% over three to six months. Details about this therapy are provided in Chapter 25.

Another exclusion is having urinary difficulties such as a slow stream, getting up at night to urinate, or urinary frequency. As describe earlier, your symptoms can be determined using the IPSS questionnaire. Many doctors will not use brachytherapy if your score is higher than 15. You still may be able to have this treatment if your symptoms improve after taking hormone therapy, a pill called an *alpha-blocker*, or finasteride or dutasteride, which shrink the prostate. Brachytherapy is seldom advised if you have undergone any surgical procedure to improve your urinary symptoms.

What Happens Before the Brachytherapy?

Brachytherapy is a two-step process. About two weeks before the implant, an anesthesiologist or nurse will evaluate you and an electrocardiogram and blood tests will be performed. These are done to make sure you are suitable for general anesthesia. A volume study is done with the same ultrasound equipment used for your prostate biopsy. This time, a catheter is placed into your penis and passed into the bladder so the urethra can be identified within the prostate. It is removed after the study is done. Measuring the prostate volume does not require an anesthetic and is completed in about 15 minutes. The information from the volume study is entered into a computer, which determines the best location to place the seeds and how many will be needed.

Some doctors use a different approach. Instead of preplanning the treatment, the number and location for your seeds is determined by a computer while you are under anesthesia. This approach is used because the size and shape of the prostate may change slightly between the time of the volume study and the day of the implant. More seeds must be ordered to do this approach and some may be wasted if they are not used. This can raise the cost of the treatment. No study has determined which approach is best so either is reasonable.

The decision about using ^{125}I, ^{103}Pd, or ^{131}Cs will be made by the doctor performing the procedure. Because no studies have proven that either one gives better results, they are all reasonable options. One difference may be the effect on urinary function.

A randomized study measured the urinary symptom scores in men assigned to receive ^{125}I or ^{103}Pd. The IPSS score was higher in the ^{103}Pd group at one month but lower at six months. The result does not mean that ^{103}Pd is a better choice. It simply shows that either you get slightly more severe side effects for a shorter time with ^{103}Pd or less severe side effects for a longer time with ^{125}I. In the United States, iodine seeds are used more often for low-risk tumors because they have the longest track record. Many doctors favor the

^{125}I for low-risk cancers and ^{103}Pd for intermediate- or high-risk cancers. You can discuss the three options with your doctor and ask which one they think is best for you and for what reason.

Beginning one week before the implant, you will be told to stop taking any drugs that can increase your risk of bleeding. The most common ones are called NSAIDS, which stands for nonsteroidal anti-inflammatory drugs. They include Motrin, ibuprofen, Naprosyn, Aleve, and Celebrex. Vitamin E also should be avoided. If one of these is taken by mistake within seven days of the procedure, you should notify your doctor right away. Do not eat or drink after midnight on the day before your procedure.

On the day of your implant, you will take an enema and arrive at the treatment center about 60 to 90 minutes before the procedure. After you change into a hospital gown, a needle will be placed in your arm to administer intravenous fluids.

How Is Permanent Brachytherapy Performed?

When it is time for the procedure, you are taken into a treatment room, transferred to a table, and put to sleep by the anesthesiologist. The staff will position you on the table with your legs elevated, cleanse the rectal area, and cover it with surgical drapes.

The procedure begins by placing an ultrasound probe into your rectum. A specially designed needle guide is attached to the probe and pushed against the perineal skin above the rectum. It has many small openings positioned close to each other that are numbered. If your doctor has preplanned the treatment, the radioactive seeds will be contained in about 40 hollow needles that have been specially ordered based on your volume study. Each needle containing the right number of seeds is inserted into a specific opening on the needle guide. The seeds are left in the prostate as the needle is withdrawn. About 50 to 120 seeds will be placed during the procedure, which usually is completed in 60 to 90 minutes.

The ultrasound probe is then removed and a telescopic instrument called a *cystoscope* is inserted into the penis and bladder to look for any bleeding or remove seeds that came out of the prostate. A catheter is inserted into the bladder and left in place while you are transferred to the recovery room. It will remain there until you're fully awake. You can go home when you are able to eat, drink, and urinate. If you can't urinate, the catheter will be inserted again and stay there for one or two weeks. Most men are able to urinate after this time.

What Happens When You Are Home?

Most activities can be resumed within one or two days after the procedure. You will be instructed to urinate into a strainer to look for any seeds coming out of the prostate.

Doctors advise avoiding or limiting very close contact with children or pregnant women until the radioactivity has mostly gone away. They can be in a room with you if they are more than 6 ft away. Close contact is safe after the radiation is nearly gone which takes about 300 days with iodine seeds, 85 days with palladium, and 49 days with cesium. One of the side effects is blood in the urine, called *hematuria*. Call your doctor if you see blood clots or you have a burning sensation when you urinate.

One month after the procedure, a computerized axial tomography (CAT) scan is performed to determine the exact amount of radiation that is being delivered to your prostate. Your PSA will be checked starting at about three months.

Temporary Brachytherapy

Temporary brachytherapy is also called high dose rate or HDR brachytherapy because the radioactive material gives off more radiation each day than the material used for permanent seed implants.

What Are the Advantages and Disadvantages of Temporary Brachytherapy?

HDR has potential advantages and disadvantages compared to permanent brachytherapy and external radiation as listed in the following tables:

Advantages of Temporary Brachytherapy

Potentially more precise delivery of radiation to the prostate

No radioactive seeds left in the body

Treatment completed in two days

No risk of radiation to other people

Disadvantages of Temporary Brachytherapy

Requires anesthesia and one or two nights in the hospital

More inconvenient than permanent brachytherapy

Limited number of centers offering procedure

Long-term results not available using HDR by itself

The primary advantage of this treatment is the potential ability to more effectively tailor the radiation to the shape of the prostate. In theory, this might cause fewer side effects. A small advantage is no radiation is left in your body after the treatment is done.

HDR brachytherapy is a much more difficult treatment than a permanent implant. It requires one or two nights in the hospital, about one week apart, two anesthetics, and four to six treatment sessions.

The biggest problem is that long-term survival information is very limited. Few men have been followed for more than 10 years. Also, no well-controlled studies have been done and most reports do not contain enough information for the results to be evaluated.

Much of the information about HDR brachytherapy for men with intermediate- or high-risk cancers has been obtained by combining it with external radiation. The same problems exist for this combination; no well-done studies have been done and long-term survival has not been reported. Doctors cannot tell if HDR brachytherapy and external radiation used together are better than either treatment alone. The bottom line is HDR has potential advantages but not enough is known to tell if it is better, worse, or the same as other options.

Who Is a Good Candidate for Temporary Brachytherapy?

Not enough information is available to say who is a good candidate for HDR brachytherapy. If you have a low-risk cancer, this treatment would appear to be much more involved than a permanent implant. The only clear advantage is being able to have close contact with a child or pregnant women immediately after it's done. The same is true for an intermediate- or high-risk tumor. If most doctors are going to recommend that you also get treated with external radiation, the benefit of a temporary implant over a permanent one seems unclear. Without more evidence showing it gives better results, this treatment probably should not be chosen at this time.

What Happens Before You Undergo Temporary Brachytherapy?

Approximately one week before the procedure, you will be examined, and an electrocardiogram and blood tests will be obtained to make sure you can safely have anesthesia. Any drugs that may cause bleeding should be stopped one week before the procedure.

How Is Temporary Brachytherapy Performed?

On the day of your procedure, you will arrive at the hospital, change into a gown, and have an intravenous line started. You are then transferred to the operating room, anesthesia is started, and your legs are placed in stirrups. The area around your rectum is washed and coated with an antiseptic. A catheter is placed through the penis and into the bladder, and an ultrasound probe is placed in the rectum. About 20 thin plastic tubes are pushed through the perineal skin and into the prostate, guided by the ultrasound. They are held in place with a flexible needle guide sewn to your skin. The anesthesia is stopped after your legs have been lowered onto the table. You are then transferred to the radiology department, where a CAT scan is performed so that the amount of radiation can be planned.

Your next stop is the radiation treatment room where you will be positioned on the table and connected to a computer-controlled machine. It pushes the ^{192}Ir wires through the catheters and into the prostate. These wires remain in position for a limited time and then are moved to a new location until the whole prostate has been treated. The setup and positioning may take more than an hour but the actual treatment is completed in about 20 minutes. You should not have much discomfort. After the machine is disconnected, you will be transferred to a hospital room where you must remain in bed with the catheters in place. No radiation is left in your body.

The following day, the treatment will be repeated one or two times and then the catheters in your skin and bladder are removed, and you can go home. Normal activities can resume in a day or two. The entire process may be repeated within a few weeks.

What Happens After Temporary Brachytherapy?

Because no radiation remains in your body when you go home, you do not have to avoid contact with children or pregnant women. You can resume all your activities immediately. A PSA level will be measured starting about three months after the implant.

The Bottom Line About Brachytherapy

Current methods of performing permanent brachytherapy have been in use for more than 15 years. Like surgery and external radiation, it is a reasonable alternative for treating localized prostate cancer despite an absence of any direct comparisons with other therapies. It also causes changes in bowel, bladder, and sexual function, which may be permanent and can alter your quality-of-life. The most appropriate candidates are those with low risk or intermediate-risk disease. It may be less suitable if you have a life expectancy of 15 years or longer because its long-term effect is unknown. Permanent brachytherapy by itself may not be a good choice if you have a high-risk tumor. Although temporary brachytherapy has some potential advantages, not enough information is available about how well it works when used alone or in combination with external radiation.

Cryotherapy or "Freezing the Prostate" for Localized Prostate Cancer

What Is Cryotherapy?

Cryo means cold or freezing, so cryotherapy is a treatment in which very cold temperatures are delivered to the prostate. Other terms often used for this treatment are *cryosurgery* and *cryoablation*. How does it work? When cancer cells are cooled to very low temperatures and then rewarmed, several things happen that eventually cause them to die. Cryotherapy for prostate cancer began in the 1960s, and the methods have greatly improved over the last 15 years, making it safer and more effective.

What Are the Advantages and Disadvantages of Cryotherapy?

The advantages of this treatment are the potential to cure your prostate tumor. All the cancer cells are killed if they are inside the prostate and they are cooled to the proper temperature. The treatment is more convenient than surgery because you are not having a major operation. It is described as a "minimally invasive" treatment and has very little blood loss. Unlike surgery or any type of radiation, cryotherapy may be repeated if the cancer is not completely eliminated. The treatment is completed in several hours as compared to external radiation, which takes six to eight weeks. It avoids having radiation in your body like permanent brachytherapy.

The disadvantages are that the technology keeps changing, so long-term survival rates using the latest machines are not known. Although it was initially promoted as having fewer side effects than other treatments, that has not been the case. Most importantly, a very high percentage of men lose the ability to have erections. The next table shows the range of reported complications from several uncontrolled studies. Because none of them is based on written questionnaires, the true rates for impotence and incontinence could be higher, which means comparing these results to other treatments may be inaccurate.

Complication	Percentage of Patients
Erectile dysfunction	49%–93% (at one year)
Urinary incontinence	1%–8%
Rectal fistula	0%–0.5%
Urethral sloughing	0%–15%

Erectile dysfunction and impotence—the terms that are used when men are unable to have an erection without medication or other aids.

Urinary incontinence—means leaking urine. It ranges from a few drops with exertion to constant dripping from the penis.

Rectal fistula—an opening in the wall allowing bowel contents to leak out. After cryotherapy, the stool leaks into the urethra and comes out the tip of the penis. Most fistulas will go away without treatment, but sometimes surgery is required.

Urethral sloughing—after cryotherapy, the prostate tissue dies and sometimes causes blockage in the urinary channel. It may resolve after placing a catheter for a few weeks, but sometimes surgery is needed to open the channel.

What Are the Results With Cryotherapy?

There are several difficulties in telling you what to expect if you choose this treatment including the following:

- No well-done studies have been performed comparing cryosurgery to other treatments.

- No studies have followed men who underwent this treatment long enough to know the survival rates at 10 or 15 years.

- The definition of treatment failure is inconsistent.

As explained in Chapter 7, randomized studies are the best way to compare different treatments and none have been done with cryosurgery. Also, the real test of every option for localized prostate cancer is how many are alive 10 and 15 years after they were treated. So far, no study has reported those results with the latest equipment. Without information about survival, doctors have reported the following results for cryotherapy:

- How often the prostate-specific antigen (PSA) level goes up, which is called *biochemical failure* or does not go up, which is called *biochemical disease-free survival*.

- The percentage of men with no evidence of recurrent disease, which is called *disease-free survival*.

- How often the cancer does not spread to other parts of the body, which is called *metastatic disease-free survival*.

One problem with using biochemical failure results to compare cryotherapy to other treatments is that different definitions are being used to tell if cryotherapy is not controlling the cancer. This list shows what has been reported in different studies:

- a PSA level greater than 0.4 ng/mL

- a PSA level greater than 0.5 ng/mL

- a PSA level greater than 1.0 ng/mL

- three consecutive increases in PSA level

- an increase of 2 ng/mL above the lowest, or nadir, PSA level

The ability of cryotherapy to treat prostate cancer will vary depending on which of these definitions is used. For example, using a PSA cutoff of 1.0 ng/mL will make cryotherapy appear more effective than using a level of 0.4 ng/mL.

Also, none of these definitions is a reliable way to predict long-term survival. It might *overestimate* or *underestimate* the success with this treatment. Some men may have a low PSA at five years yet they still could eventually die of prostate cancer at 10 or 15 years. Other men could have a biochemical failure at five years and never be harmed by their cancer. This is the reason that using PSA results to compare different treatments is not ideal. Until more results are available, however, this is the information that must be used.

How well does cryotherapy prevent the PSA level from going up? One uncontrolled study estimated the results 10 years after treatment. Men were divided into three groups based on how likely their cancer would spread if left untreated. *Low risk* means they had a Gleason score of less than 7, a PSA level no higher than 10 ng/mL, and a tumor stage of T1 or T2a. *Intermediate risk* means they had either a Gleason score of 7, a tumor stage of T2b, or a PSA between 10 ng/mL and 20 ng/mL. *High risk* means they had a Gleason score above 7, a PSA above 20 ng/mL or a tumor stage of T2c. These risk groups are often used when reporting results for different treatments.

The definition of treatment failure used in this study was a rise in the PSA level of 2 ng/mL above the nadir level.

Ten-Year Biochemical Disease-free Survival Results

	Low-risk Cancers	Intermediate-risk Cancers	High-risk Cancers
Estimated result	81%	74%	46%
Range	64%–90%	62%–83%	32%–58%

This study used statistical methods to *estimate* the results because most of the men have not been followed for 10 years. These results show why comparing different treatments is so difficult. When results are *estimated*, the true result could fall anywhere within the reported range. In the low-risk group, the estimated biochemical disease-free survival is 81%, but the real number could be as low as 64% or as high as 90%. There is no way to know the exact result. Now try to compare it with a different treatment that has exactly the same estimated result of 81% with the same range of 64% to 90%. Are these treatments equally effective or is one better than the other? An accurate answer is not possible. Although they *may* be similar, it is also possible that they *differ* by 26%. There is no way to be sure if they are the same or different. This is important to understand because most doctors who recommend cryosurgery will not explain this limitation. Many studies do not even report the range of results. The end result is you get misleading information. The truth is no one can say two treatments are equally effective without comparing them in a proper study.

Who Is a Good Candidate for Cryotherapy?

Any man with localized prostate cancer is a potential candidate for cryosurgery, providing he understands that little is known about the long-term results and he is not concerned about his sexual function. Low-risk cancers may be more reasonable to treat than higher-risk cancers. It may be most appropriate for someone who wants to avoid surgery and radiation. Men should have a life expectancy of at least 10 years and be able to undergo general or spinal anesthesia. The prostate size should be less than 50 g. Men with larger prostate glands may be able to have cryotherapy if the size can be reduced using drugs that lower testosterone for three to six months.

How Is Cryotherapy Performed?

Once you decide to have this treatment, your doctor will send you for a preoperative assessment to someone from the anesthesia department about one week before the operation. They probably will order some blood tests and perform an electrocardiogram to make sure it is safe for you to undergo anesthesia.

Cryotherapy is done as an outpatient so you arrive at the treatment center a few hours before the procedure. You may be told to have an enema before arriving. The operation is performed under spinal or general anesthesia, which should prevent you from feeling any discomfort. The details of anesthesia are provided in Chapter 11. First, you will be placed on an operating table and the anesthesia will be started. You then will be placed in the *dorsal lithotomy* position, which involves spreading your legs, raising them off the table above your head, and placing them in stirrups to expose your rectum and perineal area. This area is cleansed with an antiseptic and covered with sterile drapes.

An ultrasound probe is placed into the rectum in the same way as when you had your prostate biopsy. Next, a special rubber tube called a *urethral warming catheter* is placed through the penis into the bladder. It allows water to circulate through the urethra to keep it from getting too cold, which lowers your chance of injury. Temperature-sensing needles are placed through the skin near the rectum and into the prostate and surrounding tissues. They measure the temperature during the treatment to make sure it gets cold enough inside the prostate without cooling the surrounding tissues. Then, six to eight special "freezing" needles are placed through the skin in front of your rectum. They are guided into specific locations in the prostate using the ultrasound.

After all the needles are in position, *argon gas* is passed through the cooling needles to freeze the prostate. This creates an "ice ball," which can be viewed on the ultrasound. The goal is to cool the prostate to a temperature of $-40°C$ for several minutes and then allow the prostate to rewarm. The treatment is then repeated. Freezing the prostate twice is thought to have the best chance of killing all the cells.

Afterward, the probes and tubes are removed and a tube called a *Foley catheter* is placed into the bladder through the penis to drain the urine. The anesthesia is discontinued and then you are returned to the recovery room. The procedure usually is completed in two to three hours. After the anesthetic has worn off and you are able to drink and urinate, you will be sent home. The Foley catheter may be left in place for a few days because swelling often occurs, making it hard for you to urinate. Most men find that the catheter causes only minor discomfort.

What to Expect After Going Home

You will be advised to limit activity for several days and place ice packs in your perineal area to reduce swelling and discomfort. Some doctors will prescribe antibiotics for several days to reduce the chance of getting an infection. Do not be alarmed if you see blood at the tip of the penis or in the urine as these often occur. Both should stop within several days. If you get a fever or chills or notice blood clots in the urine, contact your doctor right away.

How You Are Monitored After Cryotherapy

Follow-up after cryosurgery can be done in different ways because guidelines have not been established. A reasonable approach is to perform a PSA test and digital rectal exam approximately every three months for one or two years and then every 6 to 12 months unless the PSA is changing. Some doctors recommend doing another prostate biopsy within the first few years because the PSA level does not always predict if cancer has been eliminated. If cancer cells are still present, the treatment may be repeated. A bone scan is done if the PSA level rises more than 10 or 20 ng/mL.

What Is Focal Cryotherapy?

Most of the cancers now being detected are very small. Doctors have questioned whether cryotherapy could be done only to the area containing the cancer cells. A potential advantage of this approach is it might cause less damage to the pelvic nerves. That way, men might have a lower chance of becoming impotent. Treating only a portion of the prostate is called focal cryotherapy or a male lumpectomy.

Who Is a Candidate for Focal Cryotherapy?

Obviously, focal cryotherapy can be done only if a small amount of cancer is present in the prostate. The challenge is to make sure that you meet this requirement. Studies have shown that taking 10 or 12 samples of prostate tissue during a biopsy often underestimates the amount and location of all the cancer. Therefore, relying on just one set of biopsies may not be enough to tell where all your cancer is located.

One study took men whose first biopsy showed a small amount of cancer on one side of the prostate. They then repeated it by performing mapping biopsies under general anesthesia. Tissue was taken every 5 mm throughout the prostate and then a map was created of every spot cancer was found. Cryotherapy then was performed only in those "positive" areas.

The success of this treatment was determined by doing another set of biopsies within a year. Of the 30 men treated, four had a biopsy that showed cancer and it was not in the previously treated location. Those four underwent repeat cryotherapy; this time treating the entire gland and the cancer disappeared. The doctors reported that 85% of the men maintained their sexual function, but they did not use written surveys to confirm these results. This means more men could have had worsening sexual function.

Although the initial results are encouraging, the study has several weaknesses. Because it wasn't randomized, these men could be doing well because their cancer was not life threatening, meaning the treatment really wasn't needed. Also, the long-term results aren't known because few men were followed for 5 or 10 years. More information is needed from carefully done studies before the true effects of focal cryotherapy are known.

How Men Are Followed After Focal Cryotherapy

Because focal cryotherapy is so new, the best way to follow men has not been established. Using PSA will be difficult for two reasons. First, the PSA level will not drop nearly as low as when the entire gland is treated because normal prostate cells are still alive and they make PSA. No level can guarantee all the cancer cells have been killed. Doctors could simply check to see if the PSA stays stable but that does not guarantee all the cancer cells have been killed. The best option may be to repeat the mapping biopsies but more studies are needed to know for sure.

The Bottom Line About Cryotherapy

Cryotherapy is an option to consider for your localized cancer, providing you understand what is known and what is not known. If your goal is to have the best chance of getting rid of your cancer, this treatment is not the right one for you. At this time, doctors do not yet know the survival results at 10 years or beyond. Cryosurgery also would not be the right choice if you place a high priority on preserving your sexual function. It might be a good choice if you have a low-risk cancer and are not concerned about maintaining your ability to have erections. Other reasons you might choose it are as follows:

- You want to avoid a major operation

- Radiation is not acceptable

- You cannot live with the anxiety of watchful waiting or active surveillance

Focal cryotherapy is an interesting idea that may have a better chance of preserving your sexual function but it should be considered "experimental" until more information is available. If you are a good candidate for active surveillance but want to do "something" rather than just watch it, then this option might be worth considering.

Hormone Therapy for Localized Prostate Cancer

Testosterone is a male hormone that normally is responsible for your hair growth, muscle development, sperm production, and sexual function. In 1941, Dr. Charles Huggins discovered that testosterone stimulates prostate cancer cells to grow. Lowering or blocking this hormone killed some of these cells and slowed the growth of others. This treatment became known as *hormone therapy, androgen ablation, or androgen deprivation* and it is explained in detail in Chapter 25.

What Are the Risks and Benefits of Hormone Therapy?

Hormone therapy initially was used to treat men with metastatic prostate cancer. Since its discovery, studies have proven that it also can benefit men with less-advanced disease. So far, however, its value in men with localized disease remains uncertain. The benefit of hormone therapy is it may stop or slow progression of the disease. Depending on how long you live, hormone therapy may enable you to avoid getting any of the other treatments and prevent the cancer from causing any harm.

Doctors who favor hormone therapy for localized prostate cancer use the following arguments:

- Early hormone therapy improves survival of men with locally advanced prostate cancer who are treated with external radiation.

- Early hormone therapy improves survival in men with cancer in the lymph nodes that was discovered after a radical prostatectomy was completed.

- Early hormone therapy for locally advanced or metastatic prostate cancer results in better survival and fewer cancer-related problems.

Some doctors also think that early hormone therapy might prevent your cancer from becoming more difficult to treat in the future. When prostate cancer cells grow and divide, some of the newly formed cells change, or *mutate*. The "parent" cells respond well to hormone therapy, but the new cells often can resist this treatment. Delaying hormone therapy might not be a good idea because it allows a greater number of resistant cells to develop and they will be harder to treat in the future.

The major risks of hormone therapy are the side effects, which affect many of your bodily functions. The list is shown in the following table along with the approximate percentage of men who are affected.

Known Side Effects of Hormone Therapy	Results
Hot flashes	21%–73%
Decreased sex drive	40%–95%
Problems with sexual function	50%–80%
Decreased muscle mass	1%–4% (average loss)
Weight gain	3% (average increase in weight in 75% of patients)
Osteoporosis (thinning of the bones)	2%–3% per year

Known Side Effects of Hormone Therapy (Continued)	Results
Bone fractures	6%–9%
Increased lipid levels: 　Cholesterol 　Triglycerides 　Low density lipoproteins	 8% 27% 9%
Decreased cognitive function (thinking, calculating, memory)	47%–69% (Progresses over time)
Anemia (decreased blood count)	90% of men have 10% drop and 13% of men have 25% drop in blood count
Fatigue	2%–18%
Breast enlargement (gynecomastia)	10%–25%

These results were obtained mostly from men treated for advanced prostate cancer but they also occur in men with less advanced disease. The majority of them survived for less than five years. Some doctors worry that little is known about the frequency and severity of these side effects if you get hormone therapy for 10 years or longer.

Three side effects in particular are worth discussing: diabetes, cardiovascular disease, and heart attacks. Uncontrolled studies suggest that hormone therapy increases the risk of the first two and may increase the risk of heart attacks in men with known heart disease. So far, however, randomized studies of men who received hormone therapy combined with radiation have not found an increase in these risks. Nevertheless, the concern was important enough for the following advisory statements by the American Heart Association in 2010 (Ca, volume 60: 194–201, 2010).

- There *may* be a relation between hormone therapy and cardiovascular risk.

- There is no clear indication to refer men for evaluation before starting hormone therapy.

- Men should be referred to their primary care doctor for periodic follow-up exams.

Another concern raised by some physicians is the possibility that treating a man with hormone therapy when the cancer is localized may make the cancer worse. Laboratory studies show that when testosterone is reduced, prostate cancer cells sometimes begin to make their own nutrients. These cells are able to keep growing and become harder to treat. More studies are needed to find out if this concern is valid. Clearly, hormone therapy has significant trade-offs but these controversies cannot be resolved without a proper study.

Intermittent Hormone Therapy

More than 10 years ago, laboratory studies suggested that starting and stopping hormone therapy might be as good as or better than using it continually. This approach is called *intermittent hormone therapy, intermittent androgen deprivation,* or *IAD.* It is done by giving a man drugs for several months that lower testosterone or block its action and then stopping them after the prostate-specific antigen (PSA) level has been lowered. The treatment is restarted again when the PSA level rises. This process is repeated until the treatment is no longer effective.

The benefit of this approach is it enables men to prevent their PSA level from rising while keeping their side effects at a minimum. Some of the side effects go away as the testosterone level rises and then they return when the treatment is restarted. That can result in a better quality-of-life for some men compared to getting the treatment continuously. At this time, doctors do not know how intermittent hormone therapy affects survival, but good studies are being done and the results should be ready very soon.

Who Is a Candidate for Hormone Therapy?

Some information is available to help you decide if hormone therapy is right for you. The first consideration is your life expectancy. If it is greater than 10 years and you want to get a treatment that helps you live as long as possible, then hormone therapy is not the best choice. If your life expectancy is less than 10 years, then it might be a good option depending on your type of prostate cancer. If you have a low-risk tumor (Gleason score of less than 7, clinical stage that is less than T2b, and PSA level that is less than 10 ng/mL), then hormone therapy probably is unnecessary. You are much more likely to die of something other than prostate cancer, so why bother getting the side effects that can occur with this treatment. If you have a high-risk tumor (PSA level of more than 10 ng/mL, Gleason score of more than 7, and clinical stage T2b or T2c), then hormone therapy may be the right thing to do. This may be better than surgery or radiation if your PSA is rising quickly. It has the potential to slow down the growth of the cancer and delay it from spreading. That way, you live out your remaining years without being harmed by this disease.

What should you do if you have a high-risk cancer and your life expectancy is greater than 10 years? The answer depends on your goals. Many high-risk prostate cancers are growing outside the prostate and local therapies such as surgery or radiation may not get rid of them. Hormone therapy also is unlikely to completely get rid of the cancer but it may slow down its growth. It could be used if you are unwilling to have surgery or radiation. But if you want to have the best chance for stopping the cancer from harming you then at this time, hormone therapy would not be the right treatment.

Another factor to consider is your PSA level and how fast has it been rising. One well-done study suggested that men with a PSA doubling time less than 12 months or a PSA level greater than 50 ng/mL might benefit from early hormone therapy. If your PSA level is lower or doubling more slowly, then hormone therapy can be delayed. Suppose you have severe heart disease, can you still consider having hormone therapy? The answer is a qualified "yes." You should consult with your family doctor or cardiologist to make sure your blood pressure is well controlled and you are receiving proper medication for your cholesterol.

The last thing to consider is your quality-of-life. Hormone therapy is highly likely to take away your sex drive. It may also cause fatigue and weight gain. If you want to avoid these side effects, then a different treatment would be a better choice. You always have the option of trying hormone therapy for several months to see how it affects you. If the side effects are very bothersome, you can stop the treatment. In most but not all cases, the side effects will go away. An alternative is to consider using hormone therapy intermittently.

The Bottom Line About Hormone Therapy

So far, no studies have determined how hormone therapy affects survival in men with localized prostate cancer. For that reason, it is not recommended if you want to minimize the chance of being harmed by your cancer or maximize your survival. It does remain an option if you want to avoid the side effects of all the other treatments. It is easy to do, requiring only an injection every 3, 4, 6, or 12 months and possibly taking a pill each day. You might decide that hormone therapy is better than "doing nothing" and its side effects may be more acceptable than other treatments. By understanding the pros and cons, you should be able to decide if this treatment is right for you.

High-Intensity Focused Ultrasound

What Is High-Intensity Focused Ultrasound?

High-intensity focused ultrasound or HIFU is a treatment that uses the energy from ultrasound waves to produce very high temperatures of about 100°C or 212°F. This is the same ultrasound used during a prostate biopsy. The energy is delivered to the prostate using a different probe inserted into the rectum.

Laboratory studies have shown that HIFU can destroy cells in several organs, including the prostate gland. It has been tested as a treatment for different diseases for more than 50 years. During that time, the instruments have improved, making it safer and more effective.

What Are the Advantages and Disadvantages of High-Intensity Focused Ultrasound?

There are several reasons why HIFU is being used as a treatment for localized prostate cancer. One is that some men with low-risk cancer do not want surgery or radiation but they have trouble accepting the idea of leaving their cancer untreated even for a short time. They would be willing to accept a treatment that kills the cancer if it is easy to do and causes fewer side effects than other options.

A second reason is that HIFU is "minimally invasive," which means there are no cuts on the body. This enables men to recover quickly and possibly avoid some of the side effects of other treatments. Shortening of the penis, pain during an orgasm, or the development of a hernia theoretically should not occur with HIFU like they do with surgery but better studies are needed to be sure. Permanent urinary leakage also appears to be less common with HIFU compared to surgery. Another difference is that HIFU causes very little blood loss. Although blood transfusions are rarely needed with a robotic or perineal prostatectomy, they can occur when a retropubic prostatectomy is done. Lastly, patients do not need to be routinely hospitalized following HIFU in contrast to all men needing at least one or two nights in the hospital after their prostate is removed.

HIFU also has two potential advantages over permanent seed implantation. One is you can have close contact with children or pregnant women immediately after the treatment is done. Secondly, HIFU can be repeated if some cancer cells survive whereas repeating brachytherapy is rarely considered a good option if cancer recurs.

Advantages of HIFU over external radiation are that the treatment takes only a few hours to complete compared to six to eight weeks for external radiation and external radiation should not be repeated because of the high risk for more complications.

Although HIFU is minimally invasive, it still does have risks and disadvantages even with the latest equipment. Most importantly, the Food and Drug Administration (FDA) has not yet approved it for use in the United States. They do not believe there is enough evidence proving it is a good treatment for prostate cancer. HIFU has been available in other countries for many years. That means if you want this treatment now, it must be done in another country. Some US doctors are performing HIFU by taking their patients to treatment centers in Canada, Mexico, or the Bahamas. You also can contact one of those centers directly and arrange to have it performed by their doctors. The problem, of course, is that Medicare and most insurance companies will not pay for it so it could be very costly for you. The current fee ranges from $10,000 to $25,000 per treatment. If the cancer is not cured and the procedure has to be repeated, you will have to pay for it again.

HIFU is not suitable for all men with localized prostate cancer. It is not recommended if your prostate volume is greater than 40 cc unless hormone therapy is able to shrink it. HIFU cannot be done if you have a colostomy and your rectum is no longer open.

Despite its use for many years around the world, the true rates of side effects have not been determined using written surveys. Without them, a valid comparison between HIFU and other treatments cannot be done and telling you the true odds of getting side effects is difficult to do. Although it has been marketed as having a low chance of impotence, that is not the case. It now appears that side effects are more common than expected. Some of the side effects being reported are shown in the table followed by an explanation of them.

Complications of High-Intensity Focused Ultrasound	Frequency of Side Effects
Retrograde ejaculation	More than 90%
Impotence	20%–77%
Urinary obstruction	10%–20%
Urinary infections	7%–15%
Urethral stricture	3%–9%
Rectal fistula	0.5%–2.0%
Urinary incontinence	0%–2%

Retrograde ejaculation—the absence of fluid coming out through the tip of the penis after an orgasm. Instead, it goes into the bladder and comes out when you urinate. Many men say that retrograde ejaculation decreases their pleasure during sexual activity. There is no good treatment and usually it will be permanent.

Impotence—the inability to have an erection, which may be permanent. Not enough information is available to know the percentage of men who function normally after HIFU or require some treatment to improve erections.

Urinary obstruction—following HIFU, patients usually have a catheter left inside their bladder for about two weeks because of difficulty urinating. The catheter is placed either through the penis or through the belly. After the catheter is removed, some men still will have difficulty urinating, which requires another catheter replaced. Approximately 10% to 20% of men have difficulty urinating and need some treatment. To avoid this problem, some doctors are doing a *transurethral resection of the prostate* or TURP. This operation removes prostate tissue that could block the urine. It is done immediately before the HIFU procedure under the same anesthetic.

Urinary infections—although an antibiotic is given before the HIFU is done, some men still get an infection, which usually responds to more antibiotics.

Urethral stricture—a scar that forms in the urinary tract. A plastic tube called a dilator or a metal instrument, called a *sound*, is passed into the penis and through the scar to stretch it. Another option is a minor operation called a *visual internal urethrotomy (VIU)* in which a telescope is passed into the urethra and an attached knife can cut the scar. Some patients require these treatments more than once.

Rectal fistula—because the rectum is very close to the back of the prostate, intense heat can cause damage to the rectal wall leading to a small opening called a *fistula*. It may close on its own without any treatment but in some cases may require an operation.

Urinary incontinence—some men leak urine following HIFU, which gradually goes away in most cases. A small number are left with severe and permanent leakage, which may require surgery. It is explained in Chapter 19.

What Are the Results With High-Intensity Focused Ultrasound?

Probably the most important question is whether this treatment is as effective as other treatments for localized prostate cancer. The best answer is that HIFU is a "work in progress." Although the new instruments have been used to treat men in other countries for more than 10 years, no published study has reported 10-year survival results or even 10-year recurrence rates. Most of the studies only estimate what happens in three to five years, which is not a reliable way to tell if it is effective. As discussed in Chapter 7, comparing treatments at less than 10 years is very unreliable. Most men managed by watchful waiting and active surveillance do just as well in that time. The bottom line is that an accurate comparison between HIFU and surgery or radiation is not possible at this time.

Because long-term survival results are not available, some weak studies have reported post-HIFU biopsy results and serial prostate-specific antigen (PSA) measurements. The results are inconsistent, with cancer detected in 8% to 30% of the biopsies. The reasons for this wide range are the following:

- Many men did not get a repeat biopsy.

- Only six samples were obtained in some reports, which is more likely to miss some cancers.

- If a patient had a positive biopsy after the first HIFU but a negative biopsy after the procedure was repeated, the first biopsy was not counted. This underestimates the true failure rate.

The accuracy of evaluating HIFU using PSA levels is also questionable because most studies report results for patients followed less than five years. Short-term PSA results can be as misleading as short-term survival rates because it may overestimate how often the cancer has been eliminated. Another problem with reporting PSA results is that different definitions have been used to define whether the treatment has been successful including the following:

- any detectable PSA

- a PSA greater than 0.2 ng/mL

- a PSA greater than 0.5 ng/mL

- a PSA greater than 1.0 ng/mL

- an increase of 2 ng/mL above the nadir (lowest value) PSA reached

Because HIFU is supposed to destroy all the cells in the prostate, critics argue that the PSA should drop near zero. Some studies show these levels being reached in only 50% to 70% of men getting this treatment. One study found that if the lowest PSA level was between 0.2 and 1.0 ng/mL, 30% had their cancer recur. The bottom line is more information is needed before you can be told about the true effectiveness of this treatment.

How Is High-Intensity Focused Ultrasound Performed?

On the night before and the morning of the HIFU treatment, you will take an enema to clean the rectum. HIFU is performed under a general or spinal anesthetic to prevent you from moving or having pain during the procedure. After proper positioning on a table and administering the anesthetic, the HIFU probe is inserted into the rectum. This probe is similar to the ultrasound probe used to perform your biopsy except it also can focus the sound waves to a single point. After it is inserted, pictures are taken and recorded by a computer, which then creates a treatment plan.

The procedure begins by sending a pulse of energy through the probe, generating intense heat that destroys several grams of prostate tissue. After one area is treated, the probe is focused on a different area until the entire prostate has been treated. The procedure is completed in approximately two to four hours depending on the size of your prostate and whether a TURP also will be performed.

At the end of the procedure, a catheter is inserted into the bladder either through the abdomen or through the penis. It remains in place for one to two weeks and then is removed. Before going home, you will be taught how to place a catheter into the penis in case you have difficulty urinating. You can leave after recovering from the anesthetic.

Two machines currently in use are called the *Sonablate* 500 and *Ablatherm* devices. They both were developed approximately in 2000. The Sonablate 500 does have a theoretical advantage over the Ablatherm instrument. The doctor can see the prostate with the ultrasound and perform the treatment at the same time. The Ablatherm device requires that the ultrasound be performed first. The pictures taken are fed into a computer that plans the treatment. The actual treatment cannot be visualized while it is occurring. This might permit better control with the Sonablate 500 device, but no study has compared the two. Until then, either is a reasonable option.

Monitoring Patients After High-Intensity Focused Ultrasound

Because HIFU is still evolving, no one has determined the optimal timing of follow-up visits. In many of the published reports from other countries, PSA tests are done about every three months for two years. Most patients reach their nadir PSA (lowest level) within six months, which is below 0.5 ng/mL in most patients. Many surgeons also recommend performing a biopsy about three months after the procedure. If the biopsy does find cancer, you will be encouraged to have the procedure repeated or to undergo some other therapy. If the biopsy is negative, you will continue to be monitored by a PSA and digital exam.

The Bottom Line About High-Intensity Focused Ultrasound

When you weigh all your options, be aware that there simply isn't enough information to know how well HIFU works long term. Keep this in mind if you read or hear testimonials from men who have had this treatment within the past few years, consult with doctors who perform it or visit online Web sites that promote it. They all have biases favoring HIFU and *may* not present all the information accurately. Men followed for less than 10 years may appear to be doing well after HIFU not because the treatment was effective but rather because their cancer was not dangerous. Without longer follow-up or better studies, you will not know what to expect from HIFU. Studies are underway in the United States, but until they are completed, the following "Key Point" most accurately summarizes the status of HIFU at this time.

KEY POINT

Although the concept of HIFU seems appealing, the current information is inadequate to determine if HIFU is an effective treatment for localized prostate cancer with long-term survival and quality-of-life comparable to surgery or radiation.

Hopefully, more information will become available in the next few years.

How to Decide Which Treatment Is Right for You?

At this point, you may have read every chapter on managing localized prostate cancer and are no closer to knowing what to do. You understand the pros and cons of each option and may think that every one has something appealing but also things you do not like. You and your family may have been disappointed to find out that only one good study has ever been done comparing any of the options and the results do not give you the information you need to make your choice. Now it's "crunch" time and you have to decide "which treatment is right for me?" Although it may feel like a purely emotional decision, you still can be objective. That begins by reviewing what you have read. The following table shows the strengths, weaknesses, and optimal patients for every option.

Summary of Treatment Options

Treatment Options	Strengths	Weaknesses	Optimal Patients
Watchful waiting	—Avoid side effects of treatment	—Could result in shortened survival or developing metastatic disease —May lead to missed opportunity for cure —Psychologically stressful	—Low-risk and intermediate-risk tumors —Life expectancy less than 10 years —Quality-of-life is highest priority
Active surveillance	—More than 50% of patients may avoid treatment for at least 10 years —Less risk than watchful waiting	—Limited information about 10-year survival results —No long-term survival results for patients getting delayed treatment —Psychologically stressful	—Low-risk and intermediate-risk tumors —Life expectancy less than 10 years —Quality-of-life is high priority
Radical prostatectomy	—Has the most information available about long-term survival results —Will cure completely localized cancer —Ideal if sexual function is not important —Safer choice for younger men	—Has immediate effect on sexual and urinary function that improves with time —Sexual function rarely the same as before surgery	—Low-, intermediate-, and high-risk tumors —Life expectancy greater than 15 years —Want immediate results —Survival matters more than quality-of-life

Summary of Treatment Options (Continued)

Treatment Options	Strengths	Weaknesses	Optimal Patients
External radiation using 3-dimensional conformal radiation therapy (3D-CRT) or intensity-modulated radiation therapy (IMRT)	—Higher doses now safer and more effective compared to EBRT —May cure the cancer	—10- to 15-year survival results not available with higher doses —Uncertain ability to control the cancer 15 years after treatment —Poor choice if bowel dysfunction present —Delayed effect on bowel, urinary, and sexual function	—Low-, intermediate-, and high-risk tumors —Life expectancy greater than 10 years —Want to avoid surgery —Survival matters more than quality-of-life
Brachytherapy	—Quick and convenient —Sexual function maintained initially —Resume normal activities quickly	—15-year survival results not available —Some side effects increase up to two years —Poor choice if urinary problems persist despite medication	—Low-risk cancers —Life expectancy greater than 10 years —Want to resume normal activities quickly
Proton beam radiation	—Theoretical advantages over 3D-CRT or IMRT	—Poor studies assessing survival or quality-of-life —10-year survival results not available —Expensive, not covered by all insurance —Treatment centers available only in a few cities	—Low- and intermediate-risk tumors —Willing to accept new treatment without knowing effectiveness

Summary of Treatment Options (Continued)

Treatment Options	Strengths	Weaknesses	Optimal Patients
CyberKnife radiation	—Theoretical advantages over 3D-CRT or IMRT —Treatment can be completed in one week	—Poor studies assessing survival or quality-of-life —10-year survival results not available —Expensive, may not be covered by all insurance companies —Treatment centers limited —No studies proving it delivers better results	—Low- and intermediate-risk tumors —Willing to accept new treatment without knowing effectiveness
Calypso tracking IMRT	—Theoretical advantages over 3D-CRT or IMRT —Should not be inferior to either of them	—No studies proving it delivers better results	—Low-, intermediate-, and high-risk tumors —Life expectancy greater than 10 years —Want to avoid surgery —Survival matters more than quality-of-life
Cryotherapy	—May destroy cancer without surgery —Treatment can be repeated	—High risk of erectile dysfunction —10-year survival results not reported —Impact on quality-of-life not assessed well —Too early to tell if as effective as surgery	—Low-risk tumors —Life expectancy greater than 10 years —Want immediate results —Sexual function not important —Not bothered by limited follow-up

Summary of Treatment Options (Continued)

Treatment Options	Strengths	Weaknesses	Optimal Patients
High-intensity focused ultrasound	—May destroy cancer without surgery or radiation —Treatment can be repeated	—10-year survival results not reported —Impact on quality-of-life not assessed well —Too early to tell if as effective as surgery	—Low-risk tumors —Life expectancy 10 years or less —Willing to accept new treatment without knowing long-term effectiveness —Want to avoid surgery and radiation
Hormone therapy	—Avoids surgery and radiation —Delays disease progression	—Side effects decrease quality of life —Impact on survival unknown —Does not kill all cancer cells	—Low- and intermediate-risk tumors —Life expectancy greater less than 10 years —Getting rid of tumor not the primary concern

How Might Treatment Affect Your Quality-of-Life?

Making a decision about treating your prostate cancer would be so much easier if none of the treatments affected your quality-of-life, but unfortunately that is not the case. Telling you what to expect is difficult without a randomized study, but one prospective study provides some useful information. More than 1,200 men were asked to complete phone surveys before and up to two years after being treated with external radiation, permanent brachytherapy, or radical prostatectomy. Before looking at the results, you need to be aware of the following limitations:

- It is only one study and different results might occur if other men were surveyed.

- The results could be affected by each man's age and health and the doctor who delivered his care.

- Not every possible complication was included in the surveys.

- Men undergoing watchful waiting or active surveillance were not included.

- The men were free to choose how they were treated so the results cannot be used to say that one treatment results in a better quality-of-life.

- Some of the men having radiation or brachytherapy also received a short course of hormone therapy.

- The men undergoing radical prostatectomy were healthier and younger than the men who chose other treatments. About one half of them were under the age of 60.

- Only about 60% of the men have completed the two-year surveys.

- Not all men had a nerve-sparing radical prostatectomy, which might explain why some men have problems with erections.

- Men undergoing external radiation had either 3-dimensional conformal radiation therapy (3D-CRT) or intensity-modulated radiation therapy (IMRT).

- Men treated with brachytherapy had either iodine 125 (^{125}I) or palladium 103 (^{103}Pd).

Despite all these qualifying statements, the information in the following tables may help you decide if one of these treatments is right for you.

Quality-of-Life Results After Radical Prostatectomy	Before Treatment	Two Months After Treatment	Two Years After Treatment
Weak urinary stream	12%	12%	4%
Urinary frequency	17%	24%	10%
Leaking urine more than once per day	4%	52%	14%
Using pads in underwear	1%	30%	8%
Urine leakage a moderate or big problem	2%	30%	8%
Urgency to have bowel movement	1%	5%	2%
Frequent bowel movements	1%	3%	Less than 1%
Blood in stool	Less than 1%	Less than 1%	Less than 1%
Bothered by bowel function	1%	3%	1%
Poor erections	14%	88%	58%
Difficulty with orgasms	12%	62%	42%
Erections not firm	17%	90%	64%
Poor sexual function	12%	83%	53%
Sexual function a moderate or big problem	12%	59%	43%

Quality-of-Life Results After External Radiation	Before Treatment	Two Months After Treatment	Two Years After Treatment
Weak urinary stream	13%	23%	10%
Urinary frequency	16%	34%	14%
Leaking urine more than once per day	6%	15%	7%
Using pads in underwear	1%	4%	5%
Urinary leakage a moderate or big problem	11%	30%	11%
Urgency to have bowel movement	3%	18%	16%
Frequent bowel movements	2%	16%	10%
Blood in stool	1%	3%	5%
Bothered by bowel function	3%	16%	11%
Poor erections	37%	52%	60%
Difficulty with orgasms	32%	47%	50%
Erections not firm	48%	63%	66%
Poor sexual function	34%	50%	58%
Sexual function a moderate or big problem	18%	28%	37%

Quality-of-Life Results After Permanent Brachytherapy	Before Treatment	Two Months After Treatment	Two Years After Treatment
Weak urinary stream	7%	40%	11%
Urinary frequency	11%	45%	20%
Leaking urine more than once per day	5%	13%	10%
Using pads in underwear	2%	9%	8%
Urinary leakage a moderate or big problem	8%	39%	16%
Urgency to have bowel movement	4%	19%	9%
Frequent bowel movements	3%	17%	7%
Blood in stool	Less than 1%	1%	3%
Bothered by bowel function	2%	15%	8%
Poor erections	30%	51%	51%
Difficulty with orgasms	24%	49%	45%
Erections not firm	36%	58%	56%
Poor sexual function	28%	47%	46%
Sexual function a moderate or big problem	18%	34%	30%

Take-home Messages About Quality-of-Life

What do all these numbers mean? As stated previously, they cannot be used to say that one treatment gives a better quality-of-life than the others. They do, however, help "paint a better picture" for you of what happened to other men that had surgery, external radiation, or seed implantation.

Looking at the effect on bowel function gives the following results. Men having surgery report no noticeable change either at two months or two years. An urge to have a bowel movement and the frequency of bowel movements increased two months after external radiation and brachytherapy and remained slightly more common for both treatments two years later compared to the men having surgery. Bowel function remained a moderate or severe problem for 6% of men treated by brachytherapy and 8% treated by external radiation. A small percentage of the radiated men had blood in the stool two years later. Two factors that could have influenced these results are the type of external beam used and the seeds that were implanted.

Urinary function was affected in different ways. A significant percentage of each group reported that leakage was a moderate or big problem at two months. It resolved more often in those treated with external radiation. Surgery helped about 8% of men urinate with a stronger stream and less frequency at two years. The trade-off was that 10% leaked urine more than once per day and 6% thought that urinary leakage was a moderate or big problem. Nearly the same percentage of the brachytherapy group was bothered by leakage at two years.

Sexual function was most affected by all three therapies. Before treatment, only a small percentage of the surgery group had erection problems compared to the other groups. A much greater percentage of them thought it was a problem two months after treatment. Most of the men having surgery also were affected at two years. Some men did not have a nerve-sparing prostatectomy, which may partly explain these results. If you do have a nerve-sparing operation, you are less likely to have this problem but it still is likely to be more common than after radiation or brachytherapy.

These results do not come from a randomized study, so you should not view them as exactly what to expect from these treatments. The information is intended to give you some *estimates* of what can happen with each of these treatments. Quality-of-life results are not yet available for the other options discussed in the last few chapters. That means you will have to ask the doctor offering those treatments whether new information has become available. For now, these results provide you with a better sense about what can happen after these three treatments. Remember to ask your doctor about his or her results.

Factors to Consider as You Make Your Choice

After reading about each treatment and reviewing these tables, you may have decided to eliminate some, but not all of the options. The next step is for you to answer the following questions:

- How would you describe your personality?

- What is most important to you?

- What is your current quality-of-life?

Recognizing characteristics about yourself is an important part of this decision because some treatments may "fit" your personality better than others. For example, you may have a "low-risk" cancer and do not feel that the odds of benefitting from treatment are high enough to justify taking the risks. Also, you don't mind living with some uncertainty about what will happen to your cancer in the future. Then, either watchful waiting or active surveillance are the way to go, providing you will not be "worried sick" thinking about it all the time.

What if you are unwilling to "roll the dice," gambling with your life and cannot accept the possibility of missing out on a chance to be cured? Then watchful waiting, active surveillance, high-intensity focused ultrasound (HIFU), cryotherapy, proton beam therapy, temporary brachytherapy, CyberKnife, and Calypso all can be eliminated. At this time, not enough is known about how these options will affect your quality-of-life or your long-term survival. This does not mean they are inferior treatments, but without more information, they would not be the right fit for you.

Perhaps you think of yourself as someone who wants immediate results. You may be most comfortable by doing everything possible to get rid of your cancer regardless of the consequences. In that case, radical prostatectomy would be the right choice for you especially if you have a life expectancy of 15 years or more. This treatment will tell you many details about your tumor and be "out of your body." With every type of radiation, you might feel anxious as you wait to see if the cancer has been eliminated. Although you could have surgery if radiation fails, the odds of getting complications would be higher. Having surgery does not guarantee you will be cured but if the cancer is truly confined to the prostate, then it has the least uncertainty of all the options. Also, it has the most information about long-term results.

Suppose instead that you cannot stand the idea of having an operation but still want the possibility of being cured. Then 3D-CRT, IMRT, or permanent brachytherapy would be a good fit. Brachytherapy is the fastest treatment to complete. It only takes a few hours and you go home the same day, but it is less optimal for a high risk cancer. Temporary brachytherapy is more inconvenient, requiring one or two nights confined to the bed in the hospital. The benefit is you go home without any radiation in your body but long-term results are limited.

Lastly, perhaps you are an "adventurer," someone who likes taking chances. You find "theoretical" benefits appealing. You also feel comfortable gambling on new treatments even though they do not have long-term results, and you are willing to accept the consequences in case they do not work. In that case, one of the newer treatments including proton beam radiation, temporary brachytherapy, CyberKnife, Calypso, cryosurgery, or HIFU may appeal to you. The bottom line is your personality should be an important part of choosing your therapy.

The second question on that list is "What is most important to you?" Is it your survival or your quality-of-life? In an ideal world, every treatment would cure your disease and leave you with the same quality-of-life you have right now. Although treatments have clearly improved in the last 20 years, those goals have not yet been achieved. No treatment cures the disease without the *possibility* of having some negative effect on your body. Each treatment has its "package" of good and bad results. Hopefully, by now you have a better understanding of those packages that includes the odds of getting side effects rather than just having them listed.

If you decide that maximizing your quality-of-life is much more important to you than your survival, then either watchful waiting or active surveillance is the right choice especially if you have a low-risk cancer. Your quality-of-life may get worse in the future as you age or if you need treatment for your cancer, but at least nothing will change right now. For now, your quality-of-life stays where it was before your cancer was detected.

Focal cryotherapy may be a better option if you do not want to leave the cancer untreated but wish to avoid the side effects of surgery and radiation. Even though doctors do not know if it will definitely stop your cancer from recurring, it *might* be a way to preserve your quality-of-life.

Around the country, concern is growing that many men are getting a treatment for prostate cancer that is not a good "fit" for them. Your goal should be to select a treatment that also is appropriate for your current health. Suppose survival is a high priority and you are unable to have an erection despite medication or a penile pump or sexual function is no longer important to you. In either case, there is no point in having a nerve-sparing prostatectomy. Why have a slightly longer operation or increase the chance that some cancer will be left behind? Just have your prostate removed along with the nerves. If your erections already are impaired but you still can have sexual intercourse, be aware that surgery will probably worsen them more than the other treatments. Perhaps you now have difficult or frequent urination. In that case, brachytherapy will worsen those symptoms more than the other options and surgery will help it improve. Lastly, if bowel problems already exist, external radiation will have a more negative effect on your quality-of-life and might not be the right choice. The bottom line is you should combine your knowledge about each option with your goals, fears, and personality to help you make this decision.

The Role of Your Partner

If you are married or have a life partner, he or she should be part of this decision too, because what happens to you will also have some effect on your partner. It should be no surprise that your partner may have different goals. Many men, particularly those younger than 60, place the highest priority on preserving sexual function but their partner places the highest priority on getting rid of the cancer. What are you supposed to do if you are strongly considering watchful waiting or active surveillance, but your partner wants your prostate removed tomorrow? There is no easy solution and certainly no "right" answer. The best advice is to continue to talk about it and make sure that your partner has the correct facts rather than just an emotional reaction. There even may be a role for a counselor to help you discuss your differences.

The Doctor's Role in Selecting Your Treatment

As you work through this process, two obvious places to turn for help are your family doctor and your urologist or radiation therapist. By now, you have already been informed about the options and probably heard a "recommendation" from the specialist. If you have been told that, "X" is the best treatment, a red flag should go up. Nothing is wrong with a doctor offering his or her *opinion*, but it should be made clear to you that it is just an opinion. You now know that only surgery and watchful waiting have been compared properly, which showed a better survival with surgery. No other study has proven that one of the treatments is better than another. For that reason, any recommendations involving other treatments is not being based on a good study proving it is best.

Increasingly, doctors are becoming more balanced, choosing to explain the pros and cons of each option and let their patients decide rather than telling them what to do. Although that may be unsettling to you, it's the most honest way to help you. Right now, doctors do not have all the answers. Do you really want them to decide when they don't know what's best? If you still would prefer them making the decision, then just ask and they will be happy to do so. Just remember that without proper studies, the best way to treat your prostate cancer will remain uncertain and the best treatment for one man is not the best for another.

You might think of asking your doctor, "What would you do if you were me?" Unfortunately, you are likely to get a biased answer. An interesting survey was done in which urologists, oncologists, and radiation therapists were asked, "What would they recommend for a 60-year-old, healthy member of their family?" Not surprisingly, nearly all the surgeons answered surgery, nearly all the radiation therapists answered radiation, and the oncologists were split. It is not very different from asking a Cadillac salesperson "What car should I buy, a Cadillac or a Volvo?" That person would have trouble staying in business if he or she recommended the Volvo.

What about getting a second opinion with another doctor? That might be a reasonable thing to do, providing you tell that person you only want an unbiased assessment of your situation and not someone else to treat you. Otherwise, the advice again might be biased.

What about asking your family doctor for advice because he or she has no particular interest in which treatment you choose? That might be helpful but only if your family doctor has all the facts you have read in this book, which is highly unlikely. Otherwise, your family doctor also may have biases. What your family doctor can do, however, is provide you with information about your current health and life expectancy, which is important to know when making your decision. The bottom line is you now have the best information available to enable you to make a decision. Making a shared decision with your physician probably is the best approach.

Should You Talk to Other Patients?

Getting more information about the different treatments from men who have gone through the experience should never be a bad thing. Just be aware that you again may get a biased answer. If you talk to someone who had an excellent response to his treatment, he is highly likely to recommend it. If he had a bad result, then the opposite is likely to happen. Basing a decision on the experience of one or two men may not be that helpful and it could mislead you. Asking someone, "Would you do the same thing again?" also is not very helpful because the question is meaningless. No one gets a second chance to do it over again. Also, men do not like to admit they made a mistake. Talking to someone who has gone through the treatment you are considering might be worthwhile. That way you get a "firsthand" idea of what might occur. The prostate cancer support groups are an excellent source to find someone, or simply ask the doctor who is going to treat you for a person to contact.

The Bottom Line About Choosing Your Treatment

No doubt, you have gone through a difficult emotional experience starting with your PSA test. First, you had anxiety worrying if it would be normal. Then, you had to wait to hear about your biopsy result. Finally, you find yourself overwhelmed trying to decide what to do. The best advice is to not panic but instead review the pros and cons of your options, answer the questions that have been laid out for you in this book, and keep in mind your goals, fears, and personality. This should enable you decide which treatment is right for you.

How to Improve Your Quality-of-Life

When your treatment has been completed, the priority can shift to improving your quality-of-life. That mostly means treating any problems that affected your sexual, urinary, and bowel function. The most important message in this chapter is that treatments are available to help you. Many doctors will not routinely ask you about specific problems. Rather, they assume that if you don't bring it up, then you are probably doing okay. You will need to alert them if anything is wrong so you can get the right treatment.

Treatment Options for Erectile Dysfunction

Erectile dysfunction is a term that means something is interfering with the ability to have a normal sexual response. That could be either a decrease in your desire, which is called libido, difficulty having erections good enough for sexual intercourse, or problems having an orgasm.

Sexual desire is affected by the male sex hormone, testosterone. The only prostate cancer treatment that directly affects your libido is hormone therapy. If that is how you are being treated, then stopping it is not a good idea because it may allow the cancer to start growing again.

If your libido is low and you are not on hormone therapy, it could be due to having a low testosterone level. The testosterone level often drops as men get older. It can be measured by a simple blood test. The best time to do it is in the morning because normally it drops in the afternoon. Doctors disagree about giving testosterone to men with prostate cancer. Some think it is a bad idea in case any prostate cancer cells are still alive in the body. Raising the testosterone level back to normal *might* make those cells grow better.

Others believe that giving testosterone is quite acceptable. They argue that even when the testosterone level is below normal, more than enough still is present in the body to stimulate any cancer cells remaining after treatment. Raising the testosterone back to a more normal level should not make things any worse. If having a normal testosterone level truly was bad for men treated for prostate cancer, then all of them would have to be castrated and no one believes that is necessary. The bottom line is no study has shown that having a normal testosterone level is unsafe for a man treated for prostate cancer.

If you are having a problem with your sex drive, ask the doctor to check your testosterone. If it is low you can be treated with a testosterone gel (*Testim or Androgel*) that is applied to the skin once a day. You must avoid bathing for six hours to allow it to be absorbed. Another option is to have pellets (Testopel) inserted under the skin in the buttock every three to six months.

A low testosterone is not the only reason for a low libido; stress and certain drugs also can cause it. For example, if you are taking an antidepressant, ask your doctor if you can stop it, lower the dose, or switch to a different type of medication that does not have that side effect. If you are stressed or depressed, seeing a therapist may help you improve.

The most common problem with sexual function is reduced erections caused by damage to the pelvic nerves or the blood vessels supplying the penis. Men undergoing radical prostatectomy, cryosurgery, or high-intensity focused ultrasound (HIFU) usually have erection problems immediately after surgery. They may get better with time, but it could take up to two years. Erections will not return after radical prostatectomy unless at least one pelvic nerve was preserved. Those who are treated with radiation or seed implantation keep their erections initially, but they may get worse with time.

A controversial practice after radical prostatectomy is called *penile rehabilitation*. It is defined as the use of drugs or devices to stimulate regular erections even if a man has no interest in having sexual activity. Some studies suggest that permanent damage develops in the penis when erections do not occur for weeks or months.

Penile rehabilitation makes erections occur, which hopefully prevents damage so erections eventually can return. Several small studies suggested a benefit to routine use of some form of treatment that created erections. For that reason, many doctors have been recommending that men take one of the drugs that increases blood flow into the penis either daily or at least three times per week. They are called *phosphodiesterase-5 inhibitors* (PDE5). Three drugs have been approved by the FDA. They are *sildenafil* (*Viagra*), *vardenafil* (*Levitra*), and *tadalafil* (*Cialis*).

One good study has been done which is changing clinical practice. Vardenafil was compared to a placebo in men recovering from a nerve-sparing radical prostatectomy. It found that the groups taking a placebo or vardenafil every day had fewer erections good enough for sexual intercourse than the group taking vardenafil only "on demand." That means it was taken only on a day when the patient was interested in sexual activity. The most common side effect of vardenafil was headache, occurring in 16% of the men. These results mean taking daily medication may not be the right thing to do. Instead, you should take one of these drugs only when you are motivated. The drug should not be used if you are taking nitrates for heart disease. More studies are likely to be done to confirm these results. At this time, doctors do not know if "on demand" is the right approach to use after other prostate cancer treatments.

Another drug that helps men get erections is called *alprostadil* (*Caverject, Edex*). It is given either by an injection through a small needle placed into the side of the penis or a small pellet (MUSE) placed inside the tip of the penis using a small applicator. Both treatments usually produce stronger erections compared to the oral drugs. The value of using them regularly after surgery or "on demand" has not been well studied. Some men who don't get a good response with injecting alprostadil, do respond well to an injection of a mixture of three drugs (*papaverine, phentolamine, and prostaglandin E-1*) called trimix.

All these options have a high rate of success, producing an erection within 5 to 20 minutes. Either the nurse or doctor will show you the proper way to use them. The main side effect with both methods is pain in the penis or bruising from the injection. A rare side effect is an erection that does not go away, called *priapism*, which requires immediate medical attention.

Penile pumps have been in use for many years as another way to help men with erection problems. They are hollow plastic tubes that fit over the penis. A vacuum is created between the penis and tube by forcing air out of the chamber. Some devices create the vacuum using a battery-operated pump and others do it by a hand-regulated pump. The vacuum pulls blood into the penis creating an erection, which is maintained by placing a band near the base of the penis. The process takes only a few minutes to complete. When the band is removed, the erection goes away.

If none of these options work or is acceptable to you, another option is to have a *penile implant* or *penile prosthesis*. These are artificial devices placed inside the penis during an operation taking one to two hours. Several options are available including semirigid or malleable rods that constantly maintain an erection or inflatable devices that create an erection when desired. The semirigid rods are adjusted into the erect position when a man wants to initiate sex. The inflatable implants are less noticeable and they allow a man to have an erection whenever he wants one. None of them produces a completely normal erection because they do not inflate the tip of the penis. Even so, they do make it possible to have intercourse. The side effects include a small risk of infection and the possibility the device will stop working. Your doctor can show you samples of each one and how they work before choosing one. Most urologists are qualified to do these operations.

After reading about these options, your first reaction may be that taking a pill is okay but the others are not. The idea of putting a needle into the side of your penis, placing something inside the tip, or using a pump or penile implant may sound unappealing. You are not the first person to have those reactions, but the truth is most men and their partners find every one of them acceptable and satisfying. You are encouraged to consider all of them as a possible solution. At least you have several choices that can enable you to resume sexual intimacy with your partner.

Improving Your Urinary Function

Apart from erectile dysfunction, the most troubling side effect of the different treatments is a change in urinary function. That can be uncontrollable leakage, called urinary incontinence, a slow or weak stream or getting up at night to urinate.

Sometimes the urine leaks during coughing, sneezing, lifting or laughing, which is called *stress urinary incontinence*. Another type of leakage is called *urgency incontinence*, which means you feel a very sudden need to urinate but can't make it to the bathroom in time and leakage occurs. Each can occur immediately or develop one to two years after your treatment. Some men have both types of incontinence.

Be aware that some things you do can make the problem better or worse. For example, drinking a large volume of fluid, especially if it contains caffeine, will increase the leakage. Also, you may not be able to hold the same amount of urine as you did before your cancer was treated. Urinating sooner rather than waiting for your bladder to completely fill can be of some help.

If your problem is urgency incontinence, the doctor can perform *urodynamic studies* to determine if your bladder is working properly. Drugs called *anticholinergics* are helpful for urgency incontinence, but they are less effective for stress incontinence. They can be taken by mouth or worn as a patch. The most common side effects are dry mouth, nose, and throat. If you have both types of incontinence, taking one of these drugs will be a part of your treatment, but it usually will not solve the problem entirely. The drugs currently available are shown in the following table.

Anticholinergic Drugs for Urinary Incontinence

Generic Name	Drug Name
Darifenacin	Enablex
fesoterodine	Toviaz
Oxybutynin	Ditropan, Ditropan XL [extended-release], Oxytrol [once-weekly skin patch
Solifenacin	VESIcare
tolterodine	Detrol, Detrol LA [extended-release]
trospium chloride	Sanctura, Sanctura XR

Urgency incontinence, urinary frequency, slowing of the urinary stream, burning, and urinating at night all can occur shortly after seed implantation. These are less common because men with urinary problems usually are told not to have this treatment. If they do occur, some doctors suggest avoiding acidic or spicy foods such as fruit juices because they may make the symptoms worse. Drugs called *alpha blockers* can improve the urine stream, reduce nighttime urination, and help empty the bladder. Rarely, an operation is needed to open up the urine channel.

Stress incontinence after radical prostatectomy can be improved by doing regular exercises called *Kegel exercises*. You can learn how to do them by urinating in the shower and practice tightening the pelvic muscles until the urine flow stops. Good studies have shown that starting these exercises either four weeks before the operation or just after the catheter has been removed can shorten the time to recovery. It also can result in better urinary control one year after the operation. Doctors suggest different schedules because no studies show one is better than another. Doing them for about 5 to 10 minutes several times per day until your continence returns should be sufficient. Be careful not to do them too often because it might cause the muscles to fatigue.

Although anticholinergic drugs are not very helpful for stress incontinence after surgery, occasionally they may be worth trying. Some doctors use a drug called *imipramine* if the other drugs are not effective. It is approved as an antidepressant, but it can help some men who have both stress and urgency incontinence.

Although uncommon, some men have very severe incontinence or their quality-of-life is greatly affected by only moderate leakage. This problem is caused by damage to the urinary sphincter. The two treatment options are either a "sling operation" or placement of an artificial urinary sphincter. The sling may be an excellent option for small to moderate leakage and the artificial urinary sphincter is better for larger amounts.

The sling procedure involves increasing the support of the urethra by covering it with a synthetic mesh. This increases the resistance, which reduces or prevents urine from leaking. The sling operation has helped more than 50% of men regain urinary control. It is done during a short operation that has few complications.

The "gold standard" with the longest track record for treating stress incontinence is a synthetic urinary sphincter made of silicone. It consists of a cuff, a balloon that holds liquid and a pump. They are put in place by doing an operation under general or spinal anesthesia. The cuff is placed around the urethra at the base of the penis by making a cut in the skin in front of the rectum and then it is filled with a liquid. The balloon and the pump are put in place by making a small cut in the skin in the lower belly. The pump is placed into the scrotum near one of the testicles. The balloon is placed underneath a muscle located near the bladder and then also filled with liquid.

When all three parts are in place, they are connected to each other by silicone tubes. At the end of the operation, the openings in the skin are closed with sutures that will eventually dissolve.

The device works in the following way. The liquid in the cuff constantly presses against the urethra preventing urine from leaking out. When a man gets the urge to urinate, he squeezes the pump several times. This forces the liquid out of the cuff and into the balloon. He then begins to empty his bladder and within a few minutes, the liquid in the balloon automatically returns to the cuff again shutting off the leakage.

The artificial sphincter is a highly successful procedure. The main risks are a chance for an infection or failure of the device to work properly. More than 80% of men get significant reduction in urinary leakage.

Not all doctors do these operations so you might not be offered one of them even if you are very bothered by leakage. To get the best result possible, you should search for a urologist who has done many of them.

Another possible side effect of the cancer treatments is the formation of a scar or stricture in the urinary channel. The symptoms are a slow stream, dribbling, or an inability to urinate. The easiest way to make a diagnosis of a stricture is to do a cystoscopic exam. This involves inserting a telescope into the penis and inspecting the urethral channel. A stricture is treated either by stretching it using special instruments or cutting the scar with a knife attached to the cystoscope. In most cases, a single treatment will solve the problem.

Treatment Options for Bowel Dysfunction

Some men treated for prostate cancer complain of problems with their bowel function that includes frequent stools, diarrhea, bleeding, and an inability to control bowel movements. These happen more often after radiation than surgery. Fortunately, the rates are dropping with greater use of 3-dimensional conformal radiation therapy (3D-CRT) and intensity-modulated radiation therapy (IMRT).

Often these symptoms are only temporary. Drugs and dietary changes can help reduce diarrhea. Avoiding fiber, spicy foods, raw fruits and vegetables, beans, whole grains, and caffeine can also help until the symptoms go away. Drinking fluids is important to avoid dehydration that occurs with chronic diarrhea. Eating smaller, more frequent meals can be helpful. In severe cases, instilling drugs into the rectum or cauterizing bleeding vessels may be needed.

Treatment for Mental Health Problems

Having prostate cancer can be a much more upsetting experience than many other illnesses. They often make you feel sick and the treatments make you feel better. With prostate cancer, the opposite happens. Before you get treated, nothing is wrong. The cancer is not causing you any symptoms and you feel well. Then you get treated and end up feeling worse than before it all started. Your sexual function may be much worse, your quality-of-life may be reduced and the relationship with your partner may be affected. These changes may be very disturbing and may cause you to become depressed. The best advice is to get counseling. Antidepressants can be very helpful even if you only need them for a short time. The worst thing is to ignore your feelings, withdraw from your partner, and try to cope on your own. Fortunately, most men find that they do improve over time.

The Bottom Line

The options available for treating your side effects keep expanding. The key is for you to inform your doctor of any problems that are affecting you. That way you can get the necessary treatment that will help improve your quality-of-life so you can resume living as close to normal as possible.

What to Do if the Prostate-Specific Antigen Rises After Local Therapy

In an ideal world, every treatment for localized prostate cancer would cure everyone. Unfortunately, that does not always occur. How do doctors know whether your cancer hasn't been cured? In almost every case, the first evidence will be a rise in your prostate-specific antigen (PSA). It can happen within a few months after treatment or even 15 to 20 years later. The good news is that treatment is often unnecessary because the cancer cells in your body aren't always harmful.

If treatment does become necessary, you have many options. The problem is that doctors aren't always sure what should be done because few well-done studies have been performed. Therefore, you will need to learn the "package" of good and bad effects of every option so you can help decide what to do.

Managing a Rising Prostate-Specific Antigen for Men on Watchful Waiting

The concept of watchful waiting means not doing anything to the tumor in the prostate but rather treating symptoms if the disease gets worse. For that reason, routine PSA testing is not usually done. After all, why check to see if the PSA level has gone up from 5 to 10 ng/mL if no treatment will be given? A rising PSA level will not predict when symptoms will develop. Still, an argument can be made to do the PSA test periodically. It will enable you to avoid performing routine bone scans. Prostate cancer is highly unlikely to spread to the bones unless the PSA level reaches 10 or 20 ng/mL.

As discussed in Chapter 25, the best time to use hormone therapy is controversial. Some doctors believe there are advantages to starting it when metastatic disease is first discovered and others argue it is better to wait. If you chose to do watchful waiting for your localized cancer, then you must answer the following questions. Are you going to do early or delayed hormone therapy? Will you start treatment when the cancer begins to spread or wait until it is causing symptoms? The answer will determine whether you should have your PSA tested regularly. If you would want early hormone treatment, then have a PSA test done yearly and begin to have a bone scan when the PSA level reaches 10 ng/mL. Your next scan can be done when the PSA doubles. If instead you would prefer to delay treatment until symptoms appear, then checking your PSA is not worthwhile.

Managing a Rising Prostate-Specific Antigen for Men on Active Surveillance

As discussed in Chapter 10, active surveillance has only been in use for about 10 years, which means it is a work in progress with many unanswered questions. The most important one is, "When should you stop active surveillance and get treated?" The PSA doubling time currently is one of the indicators being used to make that decision. Treatment is advised if the PSA is doubling in less than three years. For example, if your PSA level was 6 ng/mL in March 2008, it went up to 8 ng/mL in March 2009, and to 10 ng/mL in March 2010, then you should choose a different approach. Is it possible you don't really need to be treated? The answer is yes, but for now, doctors do not want to miss out on being able to cure you. They would rather treat some men who don't need it. This may change as more studies report results of active surveillance.

Managing a Rising Prostate-Specific Antigen After Radical Prostatectomy

The PSA level eventually will rise in about 20% to 30% of men having a radical prostatectomy. Most doctors do not consider it to be important until it goes more than 0.2 or 0.4 ng/mL. Fortunately, even if it rises above those levels, the odds of being harmed by prostate cancer are low. This is important to know so you don't panic and hurry to get treated. For example, in 2005, doctors at Johns Hopkins Hospital reported their results on nearly 400 men who had a radical prostatectomy. All of them had an increase in the PSA level of more than 0.2 ng/ml. More than one half of the men had been followed for at least 10 years without being treated. During that time, only 17% of them died from prostate cancer. So you can see that most of the time, having a rising PSA level is not dangerous.

The doctors used the results from these men to develop tables estimating the odds of dying from prostate cancer in men who have had their prostate removed (see reference 2). They used three pieces of information:

- the Gleason score from surgery

- how long after surgery the PSA level went higher than 0.2 ng/mL

- how long it took for the PSA level to double

The following table shows the results 10 years after the PSA level went above 0.2 ng/mL.

Approximate Chances of Dying From Prostate Cancer Within 10 Years of the Prostate-Specific Antigen Rising Higher Than 0.2 ng/mL

	PSA Level Takes More Than Three Years To Rise	PSA Level Takes More Than Three Years To Rise	PSA Level Takes Less Than Three Years To Rise	PSA Level Takes Less Than Three Years To Rise
PSA Doubling Time in Months	Gleason Score Less Than 8	Gleason Score 8, 9, or 10	Gleason Score Less Than 8	Gleason Score 8, 9, or 10
More than 15	N2%	4%	7%	14%
9 to 14.9	5%	10%	15%	31%
3 to 8.9	16%	32%	45%	74%
Less than 3	41%	70%	85%	99%

(Freedland et al., JAMA 2005; 294: 433–439)

To use this table, you must have all three pieces of information. The study also contains results at 5 and 15 years after treatment. If you do not know the numbers, the easiest way to get them is call your doctor's office and ask for the results. If you want to avoid any chance of getting the wrong information, then ask for copies of your pathology report and all your PSA levels since surgery. Don't be surprised if your doctor does not know your PSA doubling time because most doctors do not calculate it. The most accurate way to get it is to use one of the free Internet Web sites that will figure it out for you. Type "PSA doubling time calculator" in your Web browser and several will appear. The instructions are easy to follow.

Here are some of the key results from the Johns Hopkins study.

- A PSA level rising above 0.2 ng/mL within three years of surgery is more dangerous than one rising beyond three years.

- A PSA level that takes more than 15 months to double is far less dangerous than one doubling in three months or less.

- A Gleason score less than 8 is less dangerous than a score of 8, 9, or 10.

- The chance of dying from prostate cancer in 10 years is only 2% if the PSA doubling time is more than 15 months, the Gleason score is less than 8, and the PSA level took more than three years to rise above 0.2 ng/mL. This is without getting any treatment.

- A PSA doubling time of less than three months, a Gleason score of 8, 9, or 10, and a PSA level rising above 0.2 ng/mL less within three years of surgery is very dangerous and should be treated aggressively.

Hopefully, you fall into one of the groups with a small chance of dying from your cancer. If so, you may be comfortable playing the odds and not have anything done. That way you avoid getting a treatment that wasn't necessary. You also get to preserve your quality-of-life. You can continue to monitor your PSA unless the tumor begins to cause some problem. You should realize that there are no guidelines for deciding when you should be treated. Some men may be comfortable living with a 50% risk, but others may be uncomfortable when the risk is only 20%. You and your doctor will have to decide how much risk is acceptable and whether to be treated.

If you do decide not to gamble, then you should get additional treatment called *adjuvant therapy*. Be aware that doctors do not know for sure which, if any, treatment for a rising PSA level will lower your risk of dying from prostate cancer. For that reason, you might be willing to sign up for a study in which aggressive treatments are being tested. Otherwise, your options include the following:

- radiation therapy to the area where your prostate was located

- hormone therapy

- both radiation and hormone therapy

- radiation, hormone therapy, and chemotherapy

- hormone therapy and chemotherapy

Each has risks and benefits. The best choice depends on the location of the cancer. It could be in the *prostate bed*, which is where the prostate was located, some other place in the body, or in both places.

Radiation makes the most sense when all the cells are in the prostate bed and hormone therapy makes the most sense if the cells are somewhere else. Few doctors recommend getting both treatments because little information has been reported using that approach.

How can your doctor find out where the cancer cells are located? At this time, no test is 100% accurate. The computerized axial tomography (CAT) scan, magnetic resonance imaging (MRI), and bone scan are very unreliable, especially when the PSA level is less than 10 or 20 ng/mL. The Prostascint scan (see Chapter 5) probably is the best test available. The problem is it also has many false positive and false negative results when the PSA level is less than 5 ng/mL. A *false positive* means the test tells you cancer cells are in the body when they aren't. A *false negative* means they are somewhere in the body but the test does not detect them. In either case, the test gives you wrong information that could lead to the wrong treatment. Some studies suggest that a slowly rising PSA level with a long PSA doubling time means the cells most likely are only in the prostate bed.

Although doctors do not know for sure whether radiation for a rising PSA level will help you live longer, some things are known:

- Radiation is more successful if it is given when the PSA level is less than 0.5 ng/mL.

- Men with a Gleason score of 6 and a PSA level less than 10 ng/mL prior to surgery are more likely to have cancer recur only in the prostate bed.

- More than one half of men who get radiation will eventually have another rise in their PSA level.

- The success of radiation depends on the PSA doubling time.

Without a randomized study, doctors cannot tell whether radiation is beneficial, but it is an aggressive option for you to consider. Your best chance of benefitting is when the following arise:

- Your PSA level is less than 0.5 ng/mL.

- The PSA doubling time is longer than six months.

- The PSA level did not rise within three years of your surgery.

- You had a "low-risk" cancer before surgery was performed.

The side effects of radiation given after a radical prostatectomy were described in Chapter 11. Some studies suggest that the complication rates are not much higher compared to men who never had surgery. Another question that has not been answered is what dose of radiation should be given. Different amounts have been used ranging from 60 to 70 Gy but the best amount is not known.

Even if you have tumor cells in the prostate bed, hormone therapy is still an option, but it does have many side effects as discussed in Chapter 25. Also, no information is available about its effect on survival. Some doctors are suggesting a modified approach. Rather than lowering the testosterone in the entire body, which causes many side effects, they are using two drugs that affect testosterone only in the prostate cancer cells. One drug is called an *antiandrogen* and the other is called a *5-alpha reductase inhibitor* (see Chapter 26). Both can lower the PSA level without causing many side effects. Here again, not enough information is available to know if they prevent the cancer from spreading or prolong survival but one advantage is they may delay getting other treatments.

What should be done if you fall into the high-risk group? Those men have a PSA level going up within three years of surgery, a PSA doubling time less than three months, and a Gleason score of 8, 9, or 10. In that case, you are highly likely to have cancer that has spread, so radiation by itself makes little sense. Your options include hormone therapy alone, hormone therapy plus chemotherapy, or both of those combined with radiation. Little information is available to guide this decision. Because chemotherapy now is available that improves survival in men with metastatic disease, doctors are testing it in men with a fast-rising PSA level. Until results become available, few doctors will recommend it. If you are young and want to try everything possible, then at least have a consultation with an oncologist. If chemotherapy is not for you, then hormone therapy using combined androgen blockade (CAB) (see Chapter 26) might be a good choice. Another option is to join a research study.

Managing a Rising Prostate-Specific Antigen After Radiation Therapy

If you received radiation, the PSA level will drop as the cancer cells die. If some cancer cells survive, the PSA level eventually will rise. Fortunately, having a rising PSA level after radiation does not always indicate recurrent cancer.

What Is a Prostate-Specific Antigen Bounce?

Between 20% and 60% of men getting external radiation will have an unexpected increase in their PSA level by at least 0.2 ng/mL within a few years of treatment. This is called a *PSA bounce*. Doctors think it happens because some of the dying prostate cancer cells release the PSA contained inside them, which then gets into the bloodstream. *The good news is that a PSA bounce does not affect survival.* In fact, uncontrolled studies suggest those men who get a PSA bounce may be less likely to get recurrent cancer.

If your PSA level does increase after radiation, how will you know whether it is caused by a PSA bounce or a true recurrence of the cancer? A PSA bounce usually occurs within 18 months of finishing the radiation treatments, but it can occur even later. In most cases, the PSA level does not go higher than 1.2 ng/mL. It gradually goes back down over the next six months. For that reason, treatment should be delayed several months when the PSA first goes up to see if it will keep rising or return to its previous level. At this time, doctors cannot predict who will get a PSA bounce so you need to be aware that it can happen and be patient rather than panic.

Even if the rise is caused by cancer, many times it is not dangerous. If the PSA level is less than 1.5 ng/mL two years after radiation, only about 8% develop metastatic disease over the next 10 years.

What Is a Significant Rise in Prostate-Specific Antigen After Radiation Therapy?

What PSA level is thought to indicate the cancer has recurred? The answer to that question keeps changing. Years ago, it was thought to be the same as the value following surgery, namely, anything more than 0.2 ng/mL. Then it was changed to three consecutive increases in the PSA level. In 2005, it was modified again. It is now defined as an increase in the PSA level by at least 2 ng/mL more than the lowest level measured after radiation. This has been termed the Phoenix definition because it was decided at a medical conference that took place in Phoenix, Arizona.

Treatment Options for a Rising Prostate-Specific Antigen After Radiation Therapy

The treatment options for a rising PSA level after radiation also depend on where the cancer cells are located, which could be one of the following:

- in the prostate gland

- outside the prostate in some other parts of the body

- both inside the prostate and in other parts of the body

How does your doctor decide which applies for you? A prostate biopsy is the most accurate test for telling if cancer is still in the prostate. A CAT scan, bone scan, MRI, and prostate ultrasound are very inaccurate at low PSA levels. Most doctors will recommend a biopsy only if you would consider having your prostate removed, which is called a *salvage radical prostatectomy*. If a biopsy does show cancer, and you decide to have surgery, a bone scan usually will be done even though it is not very reliable.

Fortunately, most men with a rising PSA level after radiation will never need treatment because it is not life threatening. Doctors have discovered that the PSA doubling time is the best way to tell if a rising PSA level poses any danger although they don't agree on which number to use. PSA doubling times of 3, 6, 8, and 12 months have been used in some studies to separate men into low risk and high risk. Men with a short doubling time have a greater chance of developing metastatic disease over the next 10 years. They also have a greater chance of dying from prostate cancer.

Although more research is needed, finding out that your PSA doubling time is longer than 12 months may help reassure you that immediate treatment is not necessary. This information about PSA doubling times was obtained from men treated by conventional radiation. It is not known whether similar results will occur for men treated with proton beam radiation or higher doses of external radiation given by IMRT or 3D-CRT. If you do decide to get treated for a rising PSA level, your options include the following:

- salvage radical prostatectomy

- brachytherapy

- cryosurgery

- high-intensity focused ultrasound (HIFU)

- hormone therapy by itself or combined with one of the other options

As you might expect, no well-done studies have been performed, so the best treatment is not known.

The most aggressive option is to undergo a salvage radical prostatectomy. You should only consider it if your life expectancy is at least 10 years. Of course, your prostate biopsy should definitely show cancer cells otherwise, surgery would be the wrong treatment. You should also have a normal bone scan and a PSA doubling time of greater than six or nine months. Salvage surgery gives better results if done when the PSA level is less than 4 ng/mL and the PSA doubling time is not too fast.

If you decide to have a salvage radical prostatectomy, your best advice is to have it done by someone who has performed more than a few of them because it is a harder operation after radiation. Because those individuals are most likely to be at university hospitals, you can make a phone call and ask how many have been done.

Cryotherapy and brachytherapy are options with the potential to destroy any remaining cancer cells but limited information is available about their effectiveness and side effects. Although most men will have a negative biopsy after these treatments, the PSA level will eventually rise again in a high percentage of cases. Side effects do occur more often compared to men never having radiation. Both of these treatments can be combined with hormone therapy, but doctors do not know if that would be better than giving hormone therapy alone.

Candidates for these treatments are the same as those eligible for salvage radical prostatectomy. These are not good choices if the prostate is larger than 50 cc, previous prostate surgery was done for urinary problems, or cancer is in the seminal vesicles. Hormone therapy given for several months may reduce the size to an acceptable level.

The last option for directly treating the prostate is HIFU. Some poorly done studies have been published using this treatment, but less is known about its effectiveness than the other options. Also, it can cause many side effects. At this time, more information is needed before it can be suggested as a good option. Unless the Food and Drug Administration (FDA) approves it, you will have to go outside the country to get it done so it will be costly.

Hormone therapy may be a better option than the other choices because the cancer often recurs after those have been done. That strongly suggests cancer already was in other parts of the body. The best candidates for this treatment may be men with a fast doubling time. Good studies show better survival in men initially diagnosed with locally advanced disease that get immediate rather than delayed hormone therapy. It seems logical that the same benefit may occur from treating men with a rising PSA level after radiation. Proper testing will be needed to prove if that is true. Until then, it is a very appropriate option for you to consider.

Some doctors are using *intermittent hormone therapy* in this situation. Drugs are given to lower the male hormone until the PSA levels off and then the drugs are stopped. Getting a drug "holiday" gives you a chance to get rid of some of the side effects and improve your quality-of-life. When the PSA level begins to rise again, the drugs are restarted. This cycle is repeated until the PSA stops responding, which could take many years. Intermittent hormone therapy currently is being studied and the results may be coming soon. Until then, you might discuss it with your doctor as an "in-between" option. It avoids the side effects of local therapy and minimizes the side effects of hormone therapy while keeping your PSA in check. The bottom line is you have many options.

Managing a Rising Prostate-Specific Antigen After Seed Implantation

A PSA bounce also happens in up to 80% of men treated with brachytherapy. For that reason, doctors will wait several months before starting another treatment. The PSA level may take eight months or more before it drops back down to the original level.

If the PSA level continues to go up, then the cancer has probably recurred. The treatment options include the following:

- observation

- salvage radical prostatectomy

- external radiation with or without hormone therapy

- cryotherapy

- HIFU

- hormone therapy

The advantages, disadvantages, and results of each of these options are the same as for men with a rising PSA level after external radiation. Here too, very little is known about their effect on survival. Observation is a good choice because most men with a rising PSA level will not have any symptoms or problems from their cancer for many years, if ever. That way you can maintain your quality-of-life and avoid getting side effects from one of the treatments. If the cancer continues to grow and symptoms develop, hormone therapy can be started. Treatment at that time does not get rid of all the cancer cells, but it does slow down their growth and reduces symptoms.

The problem with delaying treatment is that some men may miss out on a chance to get rid of their cancer, which eventually could result in dying from the disease. If you want one of the local treatments, you should check to make sure that the cancer has not spread. None of the scans are reliable so the PSA doubling time may be the best predictor. If it is less than 9 to 12 months, the odds of the cancer already having spread are high and a local treatment may not be effective.

Managing a Rising Prostate-Specific Antigen After High-Intensity Focused Ultrasound

If you have been treated with HIFU and your PSA level rises, repeat HIFU can be considered along with any of the other local options. Here too, you should have a prostate biopsy confirming that cancer is still present. Most likely, you will have to pay for it again. If your goal is to get rid of your cancer, then you should select something other than doing repeat HIFU because no long-term survival results are available with this treatment.

Managing a Rising Prostate-Specific Antigen After Hormone Therapy

If you have been on hormone therapy and your PSA level begins to rise, what do you do next? One option is to sit tight and continue on the same therapy. The reason is that nothing else might happen for many years and starting a new therapy will only increase your side effects. Furthermore, no studies have shown adding another therapy will help you live longer.

A more aggressive approach will depend on which hormone therapy you have been taking. The details about that treatment are laid out in Chapter 25. Briefly, the first thing to do is make sure your testosterone is in the proper range. It should be less than 50 ng/dL. Sometimes the medication you are taking is not working properly and switching to a different drug may lower your PSA level. If the testosterone level is in the right range, the next step depends on whether you have been taking an antiandrogen (see Chapter 26). If so, then the next step is to stop it and repeat the PSA test in a month. If it goes down, then you can continue to follow your PSA level, and if it rises, then your next option is to consider a *second-line hormonal therapy* (see Chapter 27).

The Bottom Line

You may have found reading this chapter to be a little frustrating, wondering, "Why isn't there better information about each treatment?" The main reason is that not enough men have been willing to join research studies and their participation is an absolute requirement. Until those studies can be done, the best approach for you is to weigh the pros and cons of each choice and then tailor the decision to suit your specific situation. Fortunately, you have several options each with pros and cons.

IV

MANAGING LOCALLY ADVANCED PROSTATE CANCER

Radical Prostatectomy for Locally Advanced Prostate Cancer

Locally advanced prostate cancers are tumors growing outside the prostate capsule as judged by the digital rectal exam. They can be clinical stage T3 or clinical stage T4. Stage T3 tumors have grown through the prostate capsule into the surrounding tissues or they have spread into the seminal vesicles. Stage T4 tumors have grown into the bladder or the pelvic sidewall. Most men will have a staging bone scan to confirm that the cancer has not spread into the bones.

Locally advanced tumors are harder to treat than those that are localized. One reason is some cancer cells may already have spread to other parts of the body. There are too few of them to be detected when the cancer is diagnosed. Because none of the local therapies will get rid of those cells, the cancer eventually returns. Before widespread prostate-specific antigen (PSA) testing, locally advanced prostate cancers were very common. Fortunately, that is no longer the case. Less than 15% of all new cases are classified in these stages.

The role and value of radical prostatectomy for locally advanced tumors is more uncertain than for confined cancers. The reason is that only one randomized study has been done in the last 15 years and it has too many flaws to permit any reliable conclusions.

215

A radical prostatectomy performed on men with locally advanced disease is exactly the same as for men with a localized tumor. The only difference is that the lymph nodes should be removed in nearly every case. The side effects and details about the operation are contained in Chapter 11 and will not be repeated here.

Good arguments can be made for and against this treatment. Doctors who favor surgery use the following reasons. First, removing the prostate can reduce the chances of getting urinary or kidney obstruction in the future. This happens to 15% to 25% of men when the prostate is not removed. Either a surgical procedure, hormone therapy, or a combination of the two will be needed to treat those problems.

A second reason is to find out if cancer has spread to the lymph nodes. The only reliable way to know is to remove them. One good study has been done on men found to have lymph node metastases. It showed that doing a radical prostatectomy followed by immediate hormone therapy gives a better survival than doing the prostatectomy alone and delaying hormone therapy.

Another reason to do a prostatectomy is that the digital rectal exam is not always accurate. About 15% to 25% of men thought to have cancer growing outside the prostate turn out to be overstaged. This means their cancer really was localized rather than locally advanced. If surgery had not been done, they most likely would have been treated with radiation combined with more than two years of hormone therapy. The side effects of those treatments might be more bothersome than the side effects of surgery.

Lastly, even if cancer is growing outside the prostate, randomized studies show that giving radiation shortly after a prostatectomy can increase the chances for survival.

The arguments against radical prostatectomy are also valid. First, removing all the cancer is very difficult. Although it is true that some men are overstaged by the digital rectal exam, the vast majority is correctly staged. Normally, the goal of surgery is to remove a margin of normal tissue surrounding a tumor. Getting a clear margin cannot be done with most locally advanced prostate cancers. The reason is that the rectum is very close to the prostate gland and it might be injured. This means some cancer cells usually will be left behind after the prostatectomy if a man has locally advanced disease. Although it is true that giving radiation after surgery will increase the chances for survival, it only helps one out of every nine men. Thus, most men who get radiation after surgery do not benefit. Doctors believe that a better approach is to do radiation without surgery. This argument is even stronger because studies show the benefits of combining radiation with hormone therapy. Putting men through a big operation that does not cure the cancer makes little sense.

A second reason for not doing surgery is that the results might be the same if the prostate was left in place and hormone therapy was given alone. So far, no well-done study has compared these two options. Hormone therapy might be an easier approach.

Lastly, surgery is a poor choice for a man who is mostly concerned about his sexual function. The few studies reporting results after a radical prostatectomy show more than 80% have problems with erections. Saving both pelvic nerves is a bad idea for these men because it increases the chance that cancer will be left behind. Leaving one nerve can be done but the chance of regaining the ability to have erections is greatly reduced. In contrast, more men treated with hormone therapy and external radiation will get back to their baseline sexual function after the hormone therapy has stopped.

What Are the Results With Radical Prostatectomy?

Because well-done studies have not been done, the information available is less reliable. Some uncontrolled studies have followed men for many years with results being estimated using statistical methods. The results of five of these studies have been combined together into the next table.

15-Year Estimated Results After Radical Prostatectomy

No Increase in PSA	Did Not Die From Prostate Cancer	Overall Survival
38%–51%	32%–84%	37%–53%

The results are very variable because they are influenced by many factors such as the following:

- Gleason score

- the PSA level

- the health of the patients

- the percentage of men with localized disease or cancer in the lymph nodes

- the percentage of men getting external radiation, hormone therapy, or both

For these reasons, the results cannot be compared to other treatments when deciding which one is best. They are provided here to give you some idea about what has happened to men with locally advanced disease treated with a radical prostatectomy.

The side effects that can occur are no different than those occurring after surgery for localized disease. Most studies have not reported how often they occur using written surveys. You can expect the following ones to happen more often:

- sexual dysfunction

- urethral strictures

- urinary incontinence

- blood clot in the legs (deep venous thrombosis)

- formation of a fluid collection in the pelvis (lymphocele)

Sexual dysfunction will be more common because doctors usually remove one or both pelvic nerves in men with locally advanced disease. The risk of getting a urethral stricture or leaking urine probably will be higher because the cancers often invade into the bladder or urethra. Lastly, a deep venous thrombosis and lymphocele will be more common because everyone will have their lymph nodes removed. More information is definitely needed to be able to tell you exactly what to expect from this treatment.

Who Is a Good Candidate for a Radical Prostatectomy?

Despite the lack of good studies, radical prostatectomy may be a good option for you. The most important consideration is your life expectancy. Surgery is not a good choice unless you expect to live more than 10 years. Your general health also is a factor; you must be able to safely undergo anesthesia and a major operation.

The type of tumor you have will affect the success of surgery. The best results seem to occur when the PSA level is less than 20 ng/mL, the Gleason score is less than 8, and the clinical stage is only T3a. Men with these tumor traits are less likely to have cancer in the lymph nodes or need additional treatment in the future. If you are hoping to have only one treatment for your cancer, then don't choose surgery unless you have all three of them. They are not a guarantee that surgery will cure you, but your odds are better. Another factor is your PSA. If you have had several of them over the last few years and it has been going up slowly, surgery may be able to get rid of all your cancer.

Another factor to consider is how the side effects of treatment will affect your quality-of-life. Surgery would not be the right choice if you are sexually active now and hope to regain that ability after treatment. The same is true if you want to minimize your chance of having urinary problems in the future. Lastly, if bowel function is a concern, then you might choose surgery because radiation is slightly more likely to cause a problem.

The Bottom Line About Radical Prostatectomy

Good arguments can be made for and against doing a radical prostatectomy for a locally advanced cancer. Removing the entire tumor
can be done safely, but the odds of getting a complication probably
are higher than if the cancer is localized. Another disadvantage is
that surgery by itself often will not cure the disease. That means
you are highly likely to need additional therapy. You still might
decide it is right for you after learning about the other options.

If you choose to take this option, be sure to find an experienced surgeon because the operation is more difficult than for
localized disease. It also requires doing a more extensive operation
to take out the appropriate lymph nodes. Your best chance for a
good result is to choose a surgeon who has operated on many men
with locally advanced disease. Don't hesitate to ask the surgeon
how many have been done and how often complications occurred.
Radical prostatectomy is a reasonable option for locally advanced
prostate cancer, but you must understand the risks and benefits.

Radiation Therapy for Locally Advanced Disease

External Beam Radiation

Considerable progress has been made in treating locally advanced disease using external radiation therapy. In the 1980s, doctors recognized that many patients getting this treatment developed progressive disease. They concluded it often was not adequate to control these tumors. Since that time, two things have happened. Intensity-modulated radiation therapy (IMRT) and 3-dimensional conformal radiation therapy (3D-CRT) were developed that permit higher doses to be given without causing more side effects. Also, several well-done studies tested the effect of combining radiation with hormone therapy to see if better results could be achieved. This has significantly improved survival.

The goal of hormone therapy is to lower testosterone, the male sex hormone. More than 50 years ago, two doctors showed that this treatment helped men with metastatic prostate cancer. It seemed logical that it might also help men with locally advanced disease. A detailed explanation of this treatment is provided in Chapter 25.

The first important study of combining treatments assigned men to receive external radiation alone or external radiation plus hormone therapy for 36 months. An injection was given once a month to lower the testosterone level. About 80% of the men in this study had cancer outside the prostate and the others had high Gleason scores. Most of those tumors are also growing outside the prostate. That means nearly everyone in the study had locally advanced cancer. The most important results are shown in the following table.

Estimated 10-Year Results Comparing Radiation With Radiation + Hormone Therapy

Result	Radiation + Hormone Therapy	Radiation Alone
Overall survival at 5 years	79%	62%
Overall survival at 10 years	58%	40%
Died from prostate cancer	11%	31%

This study shows a large benefit from adding hormone therapy even by five years after the treatment was started. By 10 years, the estimated survival was improved by 18%. The treatment prevented many men from getting widespread disease and it lowered the chance of dying from prostate cancer by 20%. That means nearly one out of every five men benefitted from getting hormone therapy for three years. The reason the results are estimated is that not all men were followed for the full 10 years. The true benefit might be slightly lower or it could be even higher. Doctors cannot be sure without longer follow-up.

The study had some weaknesses. Nearly 10% of the men in both groups did not follow their assigned treatment. They either refused radiation or hormone therapy or did not complete a full 36 months of treatment. This should not have affected the results very much meaning radiation plus hormone therapy still would show much better survival.

Another possible problem is the study was done before 3D-CRT or IMRT were widely used. The total dose of radiation given to these men was only about 70 Gy. This could mean hormone therapy was helpful because the radiation dose was too low. If newer treatment methods using a higher dose had been used, then the hormone therapy might not have been needed. Only a new study can find out if this is true.

Lowering the testosterone did cause some added side effects. About 62% of the men noticed hot flashes. One third of the group had more than three hot flashes each day. Overall, the side effects were not very severe, but quality-of-life surveys were not used. That means more side effects probably occurred.

This study also gave doctors an opportunity to examine the effect of hormone therapy on overall health. Uncontrolled studies have suggested that hormone therapy increases a man's chance of dying from heart disease. This study showed the risk was not increased by this treatment. The bottom line is hormone therapy improves survival in men getting radiation without appearing to harm their heart.

Another well-done study compared short-term and long-term hormone therapy in men getting external radiation. It included stage T2c and T3 cancers. All the men were given hormone therapy for two months before and two months during radiation. They then were assigned to stop it or continue it for two more years. So, this study compared four months of hormone therapy to 28 months. The men getting the longer treatment were less likely to get cancer spreading to their bones. Also, men with a Gleason score of 8, 9, or 10 appeared to have better survival when they received the longer treatment. The side effects were very similar in the groups. This study also found that longer-term hormone therapy did not increase a man's chance of dying from heart disease.

Because many men do not like being on hormone therapy for a long time, another good study was done. The goal was to find out if less hormone therapy would be just as effective. Almost 80% of the men had locally advanced disease and the majority had a prostate-specific antigen (PSA) level exceeding 18 ng/mL. Everyone received hormone therapy for six months starting when radiation began. They then were assigned to stop it or get it for an additional two and a half years. So, this study compared the effect of giving hormone therapy for 6 or 36 months. It was stopped early because the group getting only six months was showing worse survival. This means that men treated with external radiation are better off getting hormone therapy for three years rather than only six months.

These three studies clearly show that the best way to help men getting radiation is to combine it with 28 or 36 months of hormone therapy. What about using this treatment even longer? One good study assigned men to get hormone therapy as long as they were alive. It also showed a better survival.

These studies raised another question. Is indefinite hormone therapy better than 36 months? Only another study can find out the answer. Giving longer hormone therapy will cause more side effects and many men choose to stop it early. For that reason, the best advice for you is to just take it for 36 months.

These studies led doctors to question the value of radiation. Is it really needed or could men do just as well by getting hormone therapy by itself? A good study was done to find out the answer. Men with locally advanced or very high-risk localized prostate cancer were assigned to get permanent hormone therapy alone or together with external radiation. The dose of radiation given was even less than the amount used with the other studies just described. The study is not yet over but so far, survival is much better if men get both treatments rather than hormone therapy by itself. The estimated difference in survival is about 20%, which means one out of every five men is benefitting from the combined treatments. Some doctors think the results would have been even better if a higher dose of radiation was used.

One concern about all of these studies is that they started more than 10 to 15 years ago. Some doctors ask whether the results would still be the same if the studies were repeated now. PSA testing enables doctors to tell when cancer is progressing much sooner than waiting for the bone scan to change. Starting hormone therapy when the PSA level begins to rise might have the same benefit as giving it with the radiation. Although that may be true, only a good study can find out. Until then, the best approach if you have locally advanced disease is to get both treatments together. The hormone treatment should be given for 28 or 36 months. The longer amount probably is better. If you get bothersome side effects, treatments are available to help so you can get the full amount. The drugs should be started either two months before the radiation or when it begins.

Despite the quality and importance of these studies, many doctors are not aware of them. Too often they recommend a shorter course of hormone therapy without any study proving it will be just as good. If you have locally advanced cancer and choose to get radiation, make sure your doctor plans to give you the right amount of hormone therapy. Otherwise you may not get the best result possible.

Some questions still remain. One is whether more radiation would lead to even better results. Uncontrolled studies suggest that higher doses not only result in fewer men getting a rise in their PSA level but it also may increase urinary side effects. Randomized studies are in progress comparing the standard dose of about 70 Gy to a dose of about 79 Gy. After 70 months, the survival rates are not different, but fewer men receiving the higher dose have gotten a rise in their PSA level. The higher amount of radiation also appears to increase the frequency of bowel complaints by about 10%. That study only includes men with localized disease so another study would be needed in men with a locally advanced tumor to know if it is also more effective. Until good studies are completed, doctors cannot tell you the best dose to use or how often side effects occur. Most men treated today get a dose greater than 70 Gy even though good studies have not proven it is better. This is being done because 3D-CRT and IMRT are safer ways to deliver more radiation. For now, you still should get 28 or 36 months of hormone therapy with your radiation even if a higher dose is used.

Brachytherapy

Another option for giving more radiation to treat locally advanced disease is to combine it with temporary or permanent brachytherapy. Doctors believe that giving a much higher dose may do a better job of killing the cancer cells. This combination has the advantage of taking less time for the treatment to be completed compared to external radiation alone. Several uncontrolled studies have been published but none of them prove this combination is a better option. The questions that need to be answered include the following:

- Is this combination better than external radiation plus hormone therapy or a higher dose of external radiation alone?

- What is the effect on men's quality-of-life?

- Is a permanent implant better than temporary brachytherapy?

- Is palladium 103 (^{103}Pd) or cesium 131 (^{131}Cs) better than iodine 125 (^{125}I)?

- Should hormone therapy be used and for how long?

One small randomized study assigned men to receive external radiation or external radiation plus a temporary implant using iridium 192. About 40% of the men had locally advanced tumors. The total dose of radiation was 66 Gy for the external radiation group and 75 Gy for the group getting both treatments. About two years after the radiation, men were supposed to have another prostate biopsy. At eight years, the results show no difference in survival. This study has several weaknesses that prevent any valid conclusions. Without better information, the value of this treatment compared to radiation alone cannot be determined.

Another option being done in some men is a combination of brachytherapy and hormone therapy. In theory, if hormone therapy helps make external radiation better, some doctors think it should also improve the results with brachytherapy? This seems very logical and it has been used in uncontrolled studies. Other doctors argue that it isn't a good option because cancer cells often have spread into the seminal vesicles and lymph nodes. Brachytherapy does not deliver enough radiation to treat those areas. Without proper studies, the value of this combination is unknown. Even so, you still may decide to do it because it is more convenient than getting external radiation. Just be aware that its effectiveness is uncertain.

One way to overcome this problem is to combine all three therapies. That means using external radiation, brachytherapy, *and* hormone therapy. This combination has also been used in a few uncontrolled studies. Some have used ^{192}Ir and others did a permanent implant of ^{103}Pd or ^{131}Cs. At this time, no information is available to be able to tell which one is best or whether any of them offers men a true added benefit. Also, no good information is available about the frequency of side effects. If you consider taking this approach, try to find out how this combination will affect your quality-of-life.

Other Methods for Delivering Radiation Therapy

Newer methods of delivering radiation therapy include proton beam radiation and the CyberKnife robotic system. Both have potential advantages, but long-term results are not available for localized disease and even less is known about treating locally advanced tumors. There is nothing wrong with choosing one of them, but again, be aware that doctors can't tell you what to expect. Until more information becomes available, you should also get hormone therapy for 28 or 36 months if you choose one of these treatments.

The Bottom Line About Radiation Therapy for Locally Advanced Disease

Much better information is available about treating locally advanced disease with radiation than any of the other options. Studies clearly show that higher survival can be achieved by combining 28 or

36 months of hormone therapy with external radiation. How this treatment compares to radical prostatectomy cannot be determined at this time. This combination has the advantage of treating cancer that is both inside and outside the prostate, which is harder to do with surgery. Other options include external radiation combined with temporary or permanent brachytherapy but not enough is known about the long-term results for it to be recommended at this time. By understanding the risks and benefits, you can decide which of these options is right for you.

Hormone Therapy for Locally Advanced Disease

The final option for men with locally advanced prostate cancer is hormone therapy. This a general term used to describe treatments that lower the male sex hormone, testosterone. It can be done with drugs either injected into a muscle or under the skin. An alternative is to remove the testicles, which is the organ producing most of this hormone. A detailed explanation of the different methods for delivering this treatment is provided in Chapter 25.

The reason to consider hormone therapy for locally advanced disease is the cancer often is more extensive than revealed by the digital rectal exam and bone scan. Some cancer cells already may have spread to other parts of the body, but doctors have no way to detect them. Surgery and radiation can't have any effect on those cells so they keep growing. Initially, the prostate-specific antigen (PSA) level goes down but then it rises again as the cells keep dividing. Hormone therapy is a better way to treat those cells.

What Are the Risks and Benefits of Hormone Therapy?

The benefits of hormone therapy are the opportunity to avoid going through surgery or radiation treatments. If some cancer cells already have spread, those treatments may be unnecessary because they don't prevent the cancer from getting worse. Getting hormone therapy enables you to avoid the side effects and inconvenience of those other treatments. Those risks seem to be higher in men treated for a locally advanced tumor compared to one that is confined inside the prostate. That means urinary control, sexual function, and bowel function may be affected, sometimes permanently. Although hormone therapy will rarely cure a man with locally advanced disease, it may do the following:

- slow down the growth of the cancer

- delay its appearance in the bones

- reduce the chance of getting urinary blockage or kidney damage

- allow you to live out your life without being harmed by the cancer

The risks of hormone therapy are that the cancer may not be controlled and then it can spread to other parts of your body. Metastatic disease also can greatly affect your quality-of-life and rarely is it curable. By choosing hormone therapy instead of one of the options, you may miss out on a chance to get rid of your tumor or avoid getting hormone therapy. This treatment also causes side effects that can greatly affect your quality-of-life. The list is shown in the next table.

Known Side Effects Of Hormone Therapy	Results
Hot flashes	21%–73%
Decreased sex drive	40%–95%
Problems with sexual function	50%–80%
Decreased muscle mass	1%–4% (average loss)

Known Side Effects Of Hormone Therapy (*Continued*)	Results
Weight gain	3% (average increase in weight in 75% of patients)
Osteoporosis (thinning of the bones)	2%–3% per year
Bone fractures	6%–9%

Increased lipid levels:
   Cholesterol
   Triglycerides
   Low density lipoproteins
	
	8%
	27%
	9%

Decreased cognitive function (thinking, calculating, memory)	47%–69% (Progresses over time)
Anemia (decreased blood count)	90% of men have 10% drop and 13% of men have 25% drop in blood count
Fatigue	2%–18%
Breast enlargement (gynecomastia)	10%–25%

Some of these side effects may be very bothersome, particularly if you are very active. The loss of your sex drive may affect your relationship unless you are already not sexually active. If you spend much time bathing at the beach or a local swimming pool, then breast enlargement, weight gain, and a decrease in your muscle mass may be a major concern. Over time, a loss of memory can be very troubling. The most common side effect is hot flashes. Drugs can be given to reduce these side effects but sometimes they will persist. Stopping the treatment does not always make them go away. Another risk is the possibility of developing a fracture due to thinning of the bones. Your take-home message is that hormone therapy is a reasonable option for treating locally advanced cancer. It does have its own set of side effects that aren't necessarily less troubling than those following surgery or radiation.

Does Hormone Therapy Increase the Risk of Heart Disease?

An ongoing debate among doctors is whether lowering testosterone increases the risk of dying from heart disease. Many poorly designed studies suggest the risk is increased by this treatment. Those studies have many reasons to question the results. In contrast, five good studies looked at the effect of using hormone therapy for 4, 28, and 36 months, or until men died. So far, not one of them has found an increased risk of dying from heart disease. Nevertheless, the concern was important enough for the American Heart Association to issue the following advisory statements in 2010 (Ca 2010; 60:194–201).

- There may be a relation between hormone therapy and cardiovascular risk.

- There is no clear indication to refer men for evaluation before starting hormone therapy.

- Men should be referred to their primary care doctor for periodic follow-up exams.

Until more studies are done, the best information available does not show an increased danger from this treatment. As a precaution, if you are worried about taking hormone therapy, the safest thing to do is to check with your family doctor or heart specialist.

What Are the Results With Hormone Therapy?

In the previous chapter, a well-done study was reviewed that compared hormone therapy alone or in combination with external radiation. Most of those men had locally advanced tumors. The study found that men getting both treatments lived longer than men getting hormone therapy alone. Hormone therapy has never been compared to surgery in a properly designed study of men with locally advanced disease. That means doctors don't know whether either one of these treatments results in better survival.

One question that has been studied is when is the best time to give hormone therapy. Should it be started immediately after the diagnosis or delayed until the cancer causes symptoms? The reason to do it immediately is the cancer cells may respond better. The advantage of waiting is to delay getting side effects.

One good study found that men who got hormone therapy right away had the following benefits. They were as follows:

- less likely to develop metastatic disease

- less likely to develop bone pain

- less likely to die from prostate cancer

Although survival was not improved, the benefits of early hormone therapy outweighed its disadvantages. The study has received some criticism but does provide good information about the best timing of hormone therapy.

Another study enrolled men who weren't suitable for surgery or radiation or they refused those treatments. Nearly one half of them had locally advanced disease. They were assigned to receive hormone therapy either immediately or when the disease caused pain or other symptoms. The study has several important results. First, survival was better in men treated immediately. At 10 years, the estimated difference in survival is about 11%. That means about one out of every nine men had an increased survival. The results are estimated because not everyone was followed for 10 years. The actual benefit could be a little smaller or much larger, and more time is needed to know for sure. Still, it does demonstrate that some men will live longer by being treated right away.

Who Is a Good Candidate for Hormone Therapy?

Although anyone with locally advanced disease can be given hormone therapy, some may be more suitable for it. If your life expectancy is less than 10 years, you may not live long enough to benefit from surgery or radiation. Hormone therapy can slow down the growth of your tumor. That will enable you to avoid surgery and radiation and live out your life without suffering from prostate cancer. You may be able to delay this treatment for several years. You also may be a good candidate if you have a high risk of developing progressive disease. One study suggested that the most dangerous tumors are those with a PSA level between 8 ng/mL and 50 ng/mL and a PSA doubling time of less than 12 months. Having a PSA level exceeding 50 ng/mL also puts you at high risk of progression. Surgery and radiation may be less likely to help you, although this needs to be tested in a proper study.

Intermittent, Continuous, and Delayed Hormone Therapy

Hormone therapy can be used in three ways:

- immediately, until it is no longer effective
- intermittently, until it is no longer effective
- delayed, until the cancer begins to cause problems

These three choices are all about the trade-offs of quality-of-life and survival. Based on the studies described earlier, immediate hormone therapy may be the best way to prolong your survival and prevent or delay the harmful effects of the cancer. Of course, the side effects of treatment can be troubling.

Intermittent therapy means getting drugs to lower your testosterone level until it becomes stable and then stopping it until the testosterone again rises. This cycle is repeated over and over again until it is no longer working. The advantage of this approach is it will give you "rest" periods during which some of the side effects may go away. A few studies suggest that quality-of-life is improved during these rest periods but the results aren't consistent. Some of them suggest that men have better sexual function during the time they are off treatment. Other studies found that over time, the testosterone is less likely to return to where it started in some men. Studies also are in progress to determine how intermittent hormone therapy affects survival. One of the challenges is in deciding the best way to do it. That means how long should it be given before it is stopped and when should it be restarted. Some doctors make this decision based on the PSA and others use the testosterone level to decide. No one has determined the best approach. Often, the patient makes this decision.

Lastly, delaying therapy has the advantage of delaying the onset of symptoms. This option may be best for a man who is sexually active, is not being bothered by any symptoms from the cancer, or has a life expectancy less than 10 years.

The Bottom Line About Hormone Therapy for Locally Advanced Disease

Hormone therapy has clear advantages and disadvantages and may be suitable for some men with locally advanced disease. Based on good studies, however, this is not the best choice if you want to maximize your survival. If that is your goal, hormone therapy should be combined with external radiation.

Making a Decision About Locally Advanced Disease

Surgery, radiation, hormone therapy, or a combination or radiation and hormone therapy, which one is right for you? Each choice has advantages and disadvantages making it hard for you to decide what to do. Having read through the last three chapters, you might feel overwhelmed and confused. You've learned about many medical studies and whether they are good or bad, but you find them difficult to digest. Now you need help putting it all together, so you can make your decision. The most important thing to sort out is, "Which option is the best fit for you?" Three things will help you get the right answer: your goals of treatment, the type of tumor you have, and your health concerns.

The place to start is with your treatment goals. Is curing this cancer your top priority or are you comfortable with just keeping it under control? Have you thought about which side effects you can live with and which ones are completely unacceptable?

Next, consider the details about your tumor. How big did it feel when your doctor did the rectal exam? Was it growing just outside the capsule or extending into the seminal vesicles or pelvic wall? What about your prostate-specific antigen (PSA) level, is it less than 20 ng/mL or more than 50 ng/mL? Has it been going up rapidly over the last few years or has it changed very little? How high is your Gleason score? Is it more than 7 or not?

Finally, how is your health? Do you have serious illnesses like heart disease or are you "fit as a fiddle"? Are you urinating without any problems or getting up several times each night to urinate? Do you have any bowel difficulties such as chronic diarrhea or blood in the stool? Lastly, how good is your sexual function? Have your erections largely gone away or are you still performing like a "30-year-old"?

The answers to all of these questions will have a great influence on choosing your treatment. You can begin with your goals. If you know that your overwhelming priority is survival, then hormone therapy would not be the right choice. It seldom is able to cure prostate cancer. Although no studies have compared surgery against radiation, good information is available on the effect of radiation and hormone therapy. The best studies show that radiation and hormone therapy together are better than either of them alone. The hormone therapy should continue for either 28 or 36 months. The radiation can be either 3-dimensional conformal radiation therapy (3D-CRT) or intensity-modulated radiation therapy (IMRT) to a dose more than 70 Gy. If you really want the most aggressive approach, then you might consider adding brachytherapy. Be aware that no studies have shown it will deliver a better result than hormone therapy combined with external radiation and it will increase your risk of side effects.

What about having surgery instead? It might be reasonable providing your tumor is not too extensive. That means it is not growing into the seminal vesicles, the PSA level is not more than 20 ng/mL, it hasn't been rising rapidly, and your Gleason score is lower than 8. Otherwise, surgery is unlikely to completely get rid of it. No information is available to tell you how surgery compares to radiation and hormones. Certainly, if you want to be cured *and* you hope to have some chance of regaining your sexual function, the odds *may be* better with radiation and hormones. To get rid of your cancer with an operation, your doctor may have to remove one or both pelvic nerves, which will greatly reduce or eliminate your chances of regaining erections.

Suppose you are more comfortable just keeping the cancer from spreading. Your life expectancy may be less than 10 years either because of your age or because of some other illness. In that case, either immediate or delayed hormone therapy would make more sense rather than surgery or radiation.

Which treatment is best for your quality-of-life? Without the right studies, the answer is unclear. External radiation would be the wrong choice if you have bowel problems, and brachytherapy would not be good if you have urinary difficulties. The biggest challenge is deciding what to do if maintaining sexual function was your highest priority. Surgery and hormone therapy could be excluded, and external radiation by itself might achieve your goals, but with a lower chance of getting rid of the cancer. You should realize that many good options exist to help improve erections if that becomes necessary. The only safe way to maintain your sexual function is to delay all treatments until it becomes absolutely necessary. This might be reasonable if you are fortunate enough to have a slower-growing cancer with a long PSA doubling time.

The bottom line is your choice should take many things into consideration. The best advice is to try to find the right fit for who you are, what kind of cancer you have, and what you hope to achieve.

V

Managing Metastatic Prostate Cancer

Primary Hormone Therapy for Metastatic Prostate Cancer

Some people get confused when cancer cells appear in a new location. They think it is a new cancer. For example, if prostate cancer cells spread into the bones, they incorrectly call it bone cancer when really it is still prostate cancer. The correct description is to say it is *metastatic* or it has *metastasized*. Prostate cancer can *metastasize* to the lymph nodes, bones, liver, lung, and brain. The bones and lymph nodes are far more common than the other sites. Prostate cancer metastases can cause many symptoms such as the following:

- bone pain

- fractures

- compression of the spinal cord with paralysis

- urinary obstruction

- kidney failure

- weakness

- weight loss

- decreased appetite

Metastatic prostate cancer causes the death of about 30,000 men each year in the United States. Fortunately, several treatments have improved men's survival and the death rate has been declining over the past few years.

What Are Male Sex Hormones?

Male sex hormones are chemicals produced in the body that are responsible for a man's secondary sex characteristics. These include sperm production, hair growth, muscle strength, and male sexual function. The most common male hormone is called *testosterone*. Approximately 95% of it is produced in the testicles and 5% is produced in the adrenal glands. The following table lists the names of the other male hormones produced by these organs.

Other Male Sex Hormones
Dehydroepiandrosterone (DHEA)
Androstenedione
Androstenediol
Androsterone
Dihydrotestosterone

What Is Hormone Therapy?

One of the properties of prostate cancer compared to all other cancers is its ability to grow in response to the male sex hormones. Dr. Charles Huggins and his colleague are credited with showing this connection and developing a treatment based on it. In 1941, they showed that lowering the testosterone level in men with metastatic disease significantly improved the symptoms. It reduced pain, improved urinary function and appetite, and helped men regain some weight. This treatment was the very first form of chemotherapy for any type of cancer and it resulted in Dr. Huggins being awarded the Nobel Prize in medicine in 1966. Today it is still the *first and best* treatment for metastatic prostate cancer.

The primary therapy for men with metastatic prostate cancer is aimed at the testosterone coming from the testicles. Several terms are used to describe this treatment including *hormone therapy, androgen ablation, hormone deprivation, androgen deprivation therapy (ADT)*, and *castration.* They all mean the same thing and any of them can be used when talking about this therapy. Hormone therapy is the term used most often in this book. Over the past 30 years, the number of hormone therapy options has increased, giving you many more choices.

The initial treatment was to remove the testicles by a quick and relatively painless operation under anesthesia called a *bilateral orchiectomy* or *bilateral orchidectomy*. Another name for it is *surgical castration.*

What to Expect From a Bilateral Orchiectomy

The operation can be performed under a local, spinal, or general anesthetic. If either the spinal or general will be used, your doctor will send you for a preoperative evaluation to make sure it is safe for you to have the anesthetic.

For at least one week before surgery, *do not take* over-the-counter medications that might increase the risk of bleeding. That includes any drug belonging to a group called *NSAIDs* or *nonsteroidal anti-inflammatory drugs* such as aspirin, Motrin, ibuprofen, Naprosyn, Aleve, and Celebrex. Vitamin E also should be avoided. If you take one of these by mistake within seven days of your scheduled surgery, notify your surgeon right away. Also, you should not eat or drink anything after midnight the day before surgery if a general or spinal anesthetic is planned.

When you arrive for surgery, you will change into a surgical gown and an intravenous line and fluids will be started. When it is time for surgery, you will be brought into the operating room and transferred onto the operating table. The anesthetic will be started and then someone will wash and shave your scrotum, coat the scrotum with an antiseptic, and then put sterile drapes around the area.

The operation begins by the surgeon making about a three-inch cut in the middle of the scrotal sac. The cut continues through the tissues until a testicle is reached. The blood vessels are tied off with sutures and then the testicle is removed. The same thing is done on the other side without making another cut in the skin. The scrotum is then closed with sutures placed under the skin. They eventually will dissolve and do not need to be removed. The entire operation usually takes less than one hour. A dressing is placed on the wound and usually ice is applied to reduce swelling.

You then will be brought to the recovery room and remain there until you are drinking liquids, passing urine and your vital signs are stable. Your activity should be limited for a few days. Ice packs can be applied to the scrotum to reduce swelling. You can shower within two days. Your doctor will recheck the wound about one or two weeks later.

A bilateral orchiectomy has few risks. The most common is bleeding under the skin, which sometimes result in a blood clot called a *hematoma*. It occurs in less than 5% of patients. In most cases, it will eventually go away without any treatment. Although an infection also is possible, it is much less common. Contact your doctor if you notice any leakage from the wound.

What Happens to the Testosterone Level Following a Bilateral Orchiectomy?

Testosterone is measured by a simple blood test. The result is expressed either as nanograms per deciliter, abbreviated as ng/dL, or nanomoles per liter, abbreviated nmol/L. The first one is used more often. Normal adult men have testosterone levels ranging from 250–800 ng/dL, which often goes down with aging. It also fluctuates every day. It is highest in the morning and lowest late in the afternoon.

After the testicles are removed, the testosterone level begins to drop, reaching its lowest level called the *nadir* within a few days. Years ago, the test used to measure this hormone was not very sensitive, meaning it could not measure very low levels. The test could tell if a blood sample contained less than 50 ng/dL, but it could not tell if the exact level was 20, 30, or 40 ng/dL. For that reason, the Food and Drug Administration (FDA) defined a level less than 50 ng/dL as the goal to reach with hormone therapy. This is called the *castrate level.*

Many years later, the test for testosterone improved making it possible to measure much lower levels. When this more sensitive test was done on men who had undergone surgical castration, the testosterone level was found to be much lower than 50 ng/dL, as shown in the following table.

Result After Bilateral Orchiectomy	Testosterone Level (ng/dL)*
Highest testosterone	30
Lowest testosterone	10
Median testosterone (1/2 of patients are above and 1/2 are below this level)	15
75% of testosterone values less than:	20
20% of testosterone values less than:	10

*Data from Oefelein, Feng, Scolieri, Ricchiutti, and Resnick. *Urology.* 2000;56(6):1021–1024.

More than three fourths of the results were less than 20 ng/dL and none were higher than 30 ng/dL.

What Is Medical Castration?

Dr. Huggins made another discovery about treating metastatic prostate cancer. The effects of surgical castration also happened to men when given a female hormone pill called diethylstilbestrol, often referred to as DES. Using a drug to reduce testosterone is called medical castration. Unfortunately, DES had one very serious side effect. About 5% of men had a heart attack when given 5 milligrams (abbreviated mg) per day. Less serious side effects were blood clots and breast enlargement.

Years later, studies were done using 1 mg and 0.25 mg per day, which did lower the heart risk, but it did not always drop the testosterone into the castrate range of less than 50 ng/dL. That led some doctors to use only 2 or 3 mg of DES per day to treat prostate cancer. Even at those doses, men still had an increased risk of heart attacks. The bottom line is that any dose of estrogen taken by mouth increases the risk of heart problems. For that reason, DES is rarely used today for the initial treatment of metastatic disease. In fact, few pharmacies now carry it.

Doctors did find out why this drug is harmful. When taken by mouth, the stomach absorbs DES. It then passes through the liver where it is changed to a different drug. The modified drug causes the heart attacks. Fortunately, doctors discovered that this side effect could be greatly reduced if estrogen was given either through a vein, into a muscle, or placed on the skin using patches or gel. All three methods are called a parenteral route of giving drugs.

They are being used in some men who get worse after primary hormone therapy and also are being tested as a first-line treatment. One well-done study compared intramuscular injections of estrogen to surgical castration or combined androgen blockade (see Chapter 26). The survival was similar and deaths from heart disease were not higher in men getting the estrogen. Parenteral estrogen has the advantages of preventing bone loss, lowering cholesterol, and avoiding hot flashes and some of the cognitive changes that occur with other drugs used to lower testosterone. The trade-off is they are more likely to cause breast enlargement. The preliminary results are very encouraging but until more studies are done, doctors cannot say if these treatments are as effective as other methods used to lower testosterone.

How Does the Body Control Testosterone?

Until the 1970s, bilateral orchiectomy and DES were the only options for lowering male hormones produced in the testicles. Then, researchers discovered a protein produced in a part of the brain called the *hypothalamus*. The name of this protein is *luteinizing hormone-releasing hormone* or LHRH. It acts on another part of the brain called the *pituitary gland* where it attaches or binds to LHRH *receptors*. You can think of LHRH and LHRH receptors as two pieces of a jigsaw puzzle that "fit" together. When this binding occurs, the pituitary gland releases another protein called *luteinizing hormone*, abbreviated as LH. It enters the blood stream and goes to the testicles where it stimulates the production of testosterone.

LHRH normally controls the amount of testosterone produced by the testicles. When the testosterone level in the bloodstream drops, LHRH production increases leading to more release of LH and then more production of testosterone. When the body has enough testosterone, LHRH goes down, less LH is released, and less testosterone is produced. This discovery led to a new way to treat prostate cancer.

Medical Castration Using Luteinizing Hormone-Releasing Hormone Agonists

Soon after LHRH was discovered, doctors began to make proteins with a slightly different chemical structure and different action than LHRH. These are called LHRH *agonists*. After one of these drugs is injected, it circulates throughout the body and goes to the pituitary gland. There, it binds to the same receptors as LHRH but it *does not* cause the release of LH. When this drug is connected to the receptors, the normal LHRH can't do its job. That leads to less

LH being released and less testosterone being produced. This causes the testosterone level to drop below 50 ng/dL into the "castrate range" within four weeks of starting this drug. This became another way to treat prostate cancer using "medical castration."

What Is a Flare Response and How Is it Managed?

Medical castration using an LHRH agonist and surgical castration have one important difference. After surgical castration, the testosterone level begins to fall immediately and reaches the nadir level within a few days. Following the first injection of an LHRH agonist, the testosterone level increases for about 10 days, and then it begins to go down. The castrate level is not reached until about 28 days after the injection. Sometimes this short-term rise in testosterone causes an increase in cancer symptoms such as more pain in the bones or more difficulty urinating. In rare cases, it can cause a spinal cord compression leading to paralysis. Any worsening of symptoms that occurs when an LHRH agonist is first started is called a *flare response*. Today, this is very uncommon, probably occurring in fewer than 5% of men with metastatic disease.

Fortunately, drugs are available that can reduce the chance of getting a flare response. The most commonly used ones belong to a group called *antiandrogens*. Although these drugs increase testosterone in the blood stream, they also prevent it from stimulating cancer cells but they are not 100% effective in preventing a flare response. In the best study done, a flare response occurred in 6% of men taking a placebo compared to only 3% of men receiving an antiandrogen called *flutamide*. Most men do not need one of these drugs unless there is extensive evidence of disease in the bones.

Three antiandrogens are currently FDA approved in the United States for use in combination with an LHRH agonist for men with metastatic prostate cancer. In alphabetical order they are *bicalutamide* (*Casodex*), *flutamide* (*Eulexin*), and *nilutamide* (*Nilandron*). Bicalutamide and nilutamide are taken once a day and flutamide is taken every eight hours. They are only needed for about 10 to 14 days to prevent the flare response because by that time, the testosterone level has dropped and the flare response stops. Side effects are very uncommon with this short course of therapy, although some men complain of diarrhea when taking flutamide. So far, no good studies have shown that one antiandrogen definitely works better than the others. Bicalutamide is used most commonly because it has fewer side effects than the other two. The FDA approval says it should be started at the same time as starting an LHRH agonist but some doctors will recommend starting it about one week before the first injection. The chance of getting a flare response is greatly reduced by about two weeks after starting the LHRH agonist.

Another drug used by some doctors to prevent the flare response is ketoconazole, which lowers testosterone levels to less than 50 ng/dL within 24 hours. It is approved by the FDA for treating fungal infections but not specifically for use in men with prostate cancer. There is no way to tell if it is better than an antiandrogen although many doctors prefer it. Ketoconazole is taken by mouth at a dose of 200 to 300 mg three times a day for about 10 to 14 days starting with the first LHRH agonist injection. Most men tolerate it without side effects, although some have nausea at the higher doses. If you are faced with the possibility of developing a flare response when starting an LHRH agonist, you should discuss these two options with your doctor and decide together which one to use.

Choosing Medical or Surgical Castration

The discovery of LHRH agonists to lower testosterone was very important for men with metastatic prostate cancer. It was safer than DES and more acceptable than having a bilateral orchiectomy. When a study was done to see which treatment men would choose if given a choice, 80% selected an LHRH agonist instead of the operation. How you are affected mentally and emotionally by a treatment is an important part of deciding which treatment is right for you.

The first LHRH agonist to be approved by the FDA required getting an injection under the skin once a day. Men were taught to do this themselves. Over time, the once-a-day drug was replaced with longer-acting ones that were given in the doctor's office. Today, LHRH agonists are administered to patients by a needle placed either *subcutaneously* (SubQ), which means underneath the skin, or *intramuscularly* (IM), which means into a large muscle.

The FDA has approved several LHRH agonists. Four of them have slightly different chemical structures from each other. To get approved, each drug had to drop the testosterone level below 50 ng/dL. The names in alphabetical order and dosing intervals are shown in the next table.

Drug Name	Chemical Name	Dosing Intervals	Made By
Eligard	Leuprolide	4 weeks, 12 weeks, 16 weeks, 24 weeks	Sanofi-Aventis
Lupron	Leuprolide	4 weeks, 12 weeks 16 weeks	Abbott
Trelstar	Triptorelin	4 weeks, 12 weeks, 24 weeks	Watson
Zoladex	Goserelin	4 weeks, 12 weeks	Astra-Zeneca
Viadur	Histrelin	12 months	Endo

You should be aware of possible confusion about the dosing intervals for each drug. Although some are being marketed using *monthly* intervals, all the studies were done using intervals measured in *weeks*. Taking a drug every six months is not the same as taking it every 24 weeks. Although not well studied, some men could have a rise in the testosterone level if the interval is based on months.

To be safe, try to schedule your next treatment by counting the number of weeks.

Having many options means you can choose a treatment interval that fits your lifestyle and circumstances. For example, if you migrate south for the winter or live hundreds of miles from your doctor, a longer-acting medication will be more convenient. If you want more frequent contact with your doctor, then you can get a shorter-acting drug.

Although you can choose the interval, you probably will be unable to choose which drug is used. Most doctors carry products made by only one or two companies for business reasons; lower prices are paid if they buy large amounts from one company. Also, the prices sometimes change. For these reasons, do not be surprised or alarmed if your doctor changes your LHRH agonist from time to time. So far, no study has shown any problem from switching drugs. Because no study has shown any one to be better, they all are reasonable options if you have metastatic disease.

The Importance of Monitoring Testosterone

Another thing to know is that LHRH agonists do not always work properly. Well-done studies show that:

- Approximately 1% to 7% of men starting an LHRH agonist do not drop their testosterone level below 50 ng/dL.

- Anywhere from 3% to 27% of men will have at least one increase in their testosterone more than 50 ng/dL even when the drug is given correctly. This is called a *testosterone escape* or a *breakthrough response*.

For these reasons, the FDA recommends checking the testosterone level in all men on these drugs. Unfortunately, most doctors do not follow this advice and instead, they just check the prostate-specific antigen (PSA). They believe that your testosterone level doesn't matter providing the PSA level drops to a very low level and stays stable. Even if they found out your testosterone level was more than 50 ng/dL, most of them would not do anything unless the PSA level increased.

Does the testosterone level matter? A few weak studies *suggest* the testosterone level is important. The first one measured at least three testosterone levels in a small number of men who had been on an LHRH agonist for several years. The study found that the cancer was more likely to get worse if the testosterone level ever went higher than 50 ng/dL. Even one increase was enough. This study is not definite proof that a testosterone level greater than 50 ng/dL is bad for you but it does suggest it is possible.

Another study measured testosterone levels in men with metastatic disease while they received an LHRH agonist. The results showed that more than one fourth of the men had a testosterone level greater than 50 ng/mL at some time after treatment. The study found that men with a higher testosterone level at six months were more likely to eventually die from their cancer compared to those with lower levels. This study also was retrospective and therefore is inconclusive.

The third one was a well-done study comparing an LHRH agonist to surgical castration. It concluded that there wasn't a significant difference in survival between the two treatments. However, a closer look at the results shows one half of the men having surgical castration lived 136 weeks compared to only 119 weeks for those getting the LHRH agonist. This difference of 17 weeks is nearly a 15% longer survival in men having surgery. The reason this difference was not called "significant" might be because the study did not enroll enough patients. One possible explanation for this difference in survival is that some men getting the LHRH agonist did not maintain their testosterone level as low as with orchiectomy. Only a larger study can prove if this is true.

One other reason to believe the testosterone level is important is that more men get very low levels after surgery than after an LHRH agonist. As shown earlier, 75% of men drop down to 20 ng/mL or lower after surgery whereas 37% to 72% of men on an LHRH agonist do not get that low.

The importance of getting and keeping your testosterone very low is not likely to be resolved any time soon. Therefore, you have to base your treatment on the best information available. A good case can be made for thinking that "lower is better." One reason is that even small amounts of testosterone can help prostate cancer cells grow. Finally, a logical argument can be made for keeping the testosterone low. Although only a proper study can test the importance of getting the testosterone level very low, it seems to make sense. That way it would be doing the same thing as removing your testicles? Until then, why not do what you can to get the best possible result, especially because you will not get more side effects? If you decide to take this approach then you should do the following:

- Make sure your doctor checks the testosterone level about two or three months after starting an LHRH agonist. If it does not drop lower than 50 ng/mL, consider trying a different drug or having surgical castration, even if your PSA level drops. Studies show that switching to a different LHRH agonist sometimes can drop the testosterone level into the right range.

- Have the testosterone rechecked once or twice each year. If the testosterone rises more than 50 ng/mL during your treatment, then talk with your doctor even if your PSA is stable. You might consider repeating the testosterone in a month, switching drugs or having surgical castration.

- If the testosterone level is lower than 50 ng/mL but much higher than 20 ng/dL, you can talk to your doctor about the pros and cons of switching your treatment to see if you can get the testosterone level lower. In some cases, this might make the PSA level go lower.

- At a minimum, talk to your doctor about this controversy when you start an LHRH agonist and make a shared decision.

The following table summarizes key points about LHRH agonist medications.

KEY POINTS ABOUT LHRH AGONISTS

1. All LHRH agonists cause an initial rise in testosterone following the first injection. This may cause a flare response in some men depending on the location and extent of the cancer. Taking an antiandrogen or ketoconazole can reduce the odds of this happening.
2. If you are receiving an LHRH agonist, ask to have your testosterone level measured between two to three months after your first injection to be sure it drops below 50 ng/dL.
3. Have your testosterone level measured once or twice each year, regardless of the PSA level because it can rise higher than the castrate level of 50 ng/dL. If that happens, then consider changing your treatment to lower the testosterone.
4. If the testosterone rises higher than 50 ng/dL, consider switching to a different medication or having the testicles removed.

Medical Castration Using a Gonadotropin-Releasing Hormone Antagonist

In 2009, the FDA approved another new drug for the treatment of advanced prostate cancer called *degarelix* (*Firmagon*). That includes men with metastatic disease and those with a rising PSA level after one of the other treatments. This medication is called a *gonadotropin-releasing hormone* (*GnRH*) *antagonist*. It works a little differently than an LHRH agonist. Degarelix binds to the receptors in the pituitary gland and immediately blocks the release of LH. This immediately stops testosterone production by the testicles. Degarelix also blocks another hormone called *follicle-stimulating hormone* or *FSH*, which normally helps sperm cells grow. That does not appear to affect prostate cancer cells.

The major advantage of degarelix compared to an LHRH agonist is that it does not cause a flare response. The testosterone level does not rise after the first injection. It means you would not have to worry about a flare response causing worsening of your symptoms during the first two weeks after starting the drug. In fact, the testosterone level drops by 90% within the first three days of getting it. One half of the patients eventually drop their testosterone to less than 9 ng/dL. Is this a better drug than the LHRH agonists? The answer isn't known because studies have not compared them. For now, they are both considered reasonable options for men with advanced prostate cancer.

Degarelix is given by an injection under the skin. The drug is injected into two places when the drug is started, each one containing 120 mg. A dose of 80 mg is then injected once every 28 days. One disadvantage of degarelix compared to the LHRH agonist is only a monthly dose is available at this time. Some men may find this more inconvenient. Another difference is about one third of men complain of pain at the injection site when the drug is started. This complaint is less common with the other drugs.

The FDA recommends also measuring testosterone regularly with this drug because 3% of men did not keep their testosterone in the castrate range. If testosterone is not maintained at that level, then you should switch to an LHRH agonist or have the testicles removed to get the testosterone into the proper range.

Intermittent Hormone Therapy

More than 15 years ago, some doctors questioned whether castration had to be a permanent treatment. They thought it might work just as well if the treatment was stopped from time to time. This idea came about because doctors thought prostate cancer cells might begin to make their own nutrients, called *growth factors*, when testosterone was absent. These might make cancer cells grow better and become resistant to treatment. They thought these growth factors would be made less often if men had intermittent rather than continuous treatment. Studies in mice supported this idea. Another possible benefit is men might have a better quality-of-life during the "rest" periods off the drug. The benefits could include a better sex drive, some weight loss, fewer hot flashes, and better energy.

The decision to stop the drugs would depend on the PSA. Once started, it would continue until the PSA dropped to a low level and then it would be stopped. The drug would be restarted when the PSA level began to rise. This process was repeated until the PSA no longer responded. The name for this treatment is *intermittent hormone therapy*.

Good studies have found that some men on intermittent hormone therapy have a better overall quality-of-life than those on permanent castration. At this time, it is not known whether intermittent hormone therapy is a good or safe approach, but good studies are underway and should be completed soon. So far, the initial results do not show any danger with this approach.

Intermittent therapy does have two possible risks. Every time an LHRH agonist is restarted, a new flare response might occur. Depending on the amount and location of metastatic disease, this could cause symptoms so an antiandrogen may be needed. Also, some doctors worry that the cancer may stop responding to treatment. Until the studies are completed, you should consider intermittent hormone therapy to be experimental. It does have potential advantages so it is an option to discuss with your doctor.

When Should Hormone Therapy Begin?

Another controversy about prostate cancer is when should hormone therapy begin in a man with metastatic disease? Should it start when metastases are first discovered even if it is not causing any symptoms, or should treatment be delayed until a man has symptoms? The reason for this debate is that few studies have been done in which treatment was delayed.

Some doctors believe treatment should be delayed because its main benefit is to reduce symptoms. If a man is not having them, then why start a treatment that can cause many side effects? It could have the effect of making someone feel worse rather than better.

Those in favor of starting it argue that the cancer is more likely to respond when less is in the body. As cells divide, changes called *mutations* can occur, resulting in their behaving differently than the cells that produced them. The mutated cells may not respond as well to a low testosterone level.

Two good studies have been done aimed at solving this debate. Patients were assigned to get immediate hormone therapy or delayed treatment. The group getting delayed hormone therapy was more likely to:

- Die from prostate cancer.

- Develop urinary blockage requiring surgery.

- Develop spinal cord compression, kidney blockage, fractured bones caused by cancer, and new metastases.

The survival was better initially and then over time, there was no difference. Still the advantages of early hormone therapy were clear for these men.

Another study enrolled men who weren't suitable for surgery or radiation or they refused those treatments. Many of them probably had very early metastatic disease, but the cancer was not causing many symptoms. Nearly one half of them had locally advanced disease. They were assigned to receive hormone therapy either immediately or when the disease began to cause pain or other symptoms. At 10 years, survival was about 11% higher in men treated immediately. This study does not prove that men with metastatic disease will also live longer, but it does support that idea.

The bottom line is that the advantages of early hormone therapy appear to outweigh the disadvantages. Therefore, *your best approach for living as long as possible and avoiding being harmed by the cancer is to begin hormone therapy when metastases are first detected.* This should be done even if you do not have symptoms from the cancer. There is a trade-off with this approach, which are the side effects that occur when the testosterone is lowered.

What Are the Side Effects of Castration and How Are They Treated?

Both surgical and medical castration does cause side effects. They can have a negative impact on men's quality-of-life and cause serious problems in some men. The most recognized ones are shown in the following table and explained in the succeeding text.

Known Side Effects of Castration	How Often They Occur or How Much Occurs
Hot flashes	21%–73%
Decreased sex drive	40%–60%
Problems with sexual function	50%
Decreased muscle mass	1%–4% (average loss)
Weight gain	3% (average increase in weight in 75% of patients)
Osteoporosis (thinning of the bones)	2%–3% per year
Bone fractures	6%–9%

Increased lipid levels:
    Cholesterol
    Triglycerides
    Low-density lipoproteins
	
	8%
	27%
	9%

Decreased cognitive function (thinking, calculating, memory)	Progresses over time

Known Side Effects of Castration (Continued)	How Often They Occur or How Much Occurs
Anemia (decreased blood count)	90% of men have 10% drop and 13% of men have 25% drop in blood count
Fatigue	2%–18%
Breast enlargement (gynecomastia)	10%–25%

Hot flashes—These are similar to the hot flashes women have when they go through menopause, but doctors do not really understand why they occur in men. Men feel sudden warmth in the face and upper body that may last seconds or a few minutes. Although they often happen several times a day, hot flashes usually are mild but occasionally can be very bothersome. Hot flashes tend to become less severe over time. The FDA has not yet approved any drugs to treat this problem but drugs used for other illnesses can be helpful. They are the following:

- *Megestrol acetate (Megace)* 20 mg two times per day
- *Gabapentin (Neurontin)* 900 mg per day
- *Medroxyprogesterone (Provera)* acetate 10 mg two times per day
- *Venlafaxine (Effexor)* 75 mg once a day

Decreased sex drive (decreased libido), impotence—Your sex drive is controlled by testosterone. As the testosterone level goes down so does your libido. Most men are still able to have erections, making sexual activity still possible. They just don't have much desire. The only way it can be treated is by allowing the testosterone level to rise, but that could make the cancer get worse. If you still want to have sexual activity and are having problems with erections, three pills are available that can help:

- *Sildenafil (Viagra)* 50 mg per day

- *Tadalafil (Cialis)* 10 or 20 mg taken every 36 hours or 2.5 or 5 mg taken once per day

- *Vardenafil (Levitra)* 10 mg per day

None of these drugs will affect your sex drive. They work by increasing blood flow into the penis.

Decreased muscle mass, weight gain—Your metabolism is partly controlled by testosterone. When the level goes down, metabolism slows and you may gain weight. Also, muscle mass decreases and fat content increases. No well-done studies have been done to show how best to treat these problems. You may benefit from meeting with a dietician to plan out a well-balanced meal with the right amount of calories for your age and body size. Also, doing weight-bearing exercises several times per week can help burn calories while protecting your bones. These include walking, weight lifting, jogging, climbing stairs, aerobics, and dancing. If regular exercise has not been part of your daily life, you should seek out a fitness expert and talk to your doctor before starting a program.

Osteoporosis and bone fractures—As men age, many develop thinning of the bones called osteoporosis. This process happens faster when the testosterone level is lowered and can lead to an increased risk of fractures. Experts recommend that you take *calcium carbonate* (500 mg daily) and a daily multivitamin containing 400 IU of vitamin D while on hormone therapy. The amount of Vitamin D in your blood can be measured by a blood test. The 2005 Dietary Guidelines recommend having a level of 80 nanomoles per liter (nmol/L). Some doctors recommend even higher levels despite no studies proving it is better. Decreased smoking and regular weight-bearing exercises can also help reduce bone loss. Also, the status of your bones should be checked with a DEXA scan (*dual energy x-ray absorptiometry*). Your best advice is to have this test done when you begin hormone therapy and then repeat it every one or two years. Most doctors do not order this test so you will have to make sure to discuss it and request one. Well-done studies have shown that osteoporosis can be treated with one of the following drugs:

- *Pamidronate disodium* (*Aredia*, 60 mg given intravenously for two hours every 12 weeks) can increase bone mineral density in men starting hormone therapy. It is not yet known if this drug will reduce the number of fractures.

- *Alendronate* (*Fosamax*, 70 mg orally once per week) was found to increase bone mineral density but its effect on preventing fractures is unknown.

- *Zoledronic acid* (*Zometa*, 4 mg given intravenously over 15 minutes every three months) was found to increase bone mineral density in men starting hormone therapy. The effect on bone fractures is unknown. Giving the drug every three or four weeks prevented cancer-related fractures in one out of nine men who failed hormone therapy.

- *Zoledronic acid* (*Zometa*, 4 mg given intravenously over 15 minutes once every 12 months) improved bone mineral density but its effect on fractures at this dose is also unknown.

- *Denosumab* (60 mg injected subcutaneously every six months) increased bone mineral density and decreased fractures over three years in men on hormone therapy. It was more effective than zoledronic acid. The FDA has approved this drug for women but it is not yet approved for men with prostate cancer. A decision is expected soon.

Some severe side effects can occur with these drugs including kidney problems, jaw problems after dental surgery, and a reduced level of calcium in the bloodstream. To avoid them, blood tests to measure your kidney function and calcium level should be done before getting each injection. If they are abnormal, medications will be recommended or the drug may be stopped. You should discuss these different options with your doctor.

Increased lipids—A low testosterone can increase your cholesterol, low-density lipoproteins, and triglycerides, which can contribute to heart disease. These changes are grouped together and called the *metabolic syndrome*. Uncontrolled studies suggest that hormone therapy increases the risk of heart disease. It may increase the risk of heart attacks in men with heart disease. So far, however, the randomized studies of men who received hormone therapy combined with radiation have not found an increase in these risks. Nevertheless, the concern was important enough for the following advisory statements by the American Heart Association in 2010 (Ca, volume 60: 194–201, 2010).

- There may be a relation between hormone therapy and cardiovascular risk.

- There is no clear indication to refer men for evaluation before starting hormone therapy.

- Men should be referred to their primary care doctor for periodic follow-up exams.

You may already have been treated for these problems before starting hormone therapy. To be safe, check with your doctor until the issue is fully resolved.

Decreased cognitive function—Some good studies have found that over time, castration results in decreased memory and a decreased ability to perform certain mental tasks such as doing calculations. These do not generally interfere with normal day-to-day activities. At this time, no studies have shown what should be done to treat this problem.

Anemia, fatigue—All adults make a protein in their kidneys called *erythropoietin*, which helps make red blood cells. Hormone therapy lowers the production of this protein sometimes resulting in a drop in the blood count within one or two months of starting treatment. A low blood count is called *anemia*, which can cause decreased energy, increased fatigue, and weakness. In those who have heart disease, it may result in shortness of breath, chest pain, and even a heart attack.

Treatment usually is not given unless symptoms occur, which happens in about 10% to 15% of men on hormone therapy. One option is to give a blood transfusion, but the blood count will drop again one to two months later. Iron supplements usually are not helpful for this problem.

A controversial option recommended by some doctors is to use a laboratory-made drug belonging to a group called *erythropoietin stimulating agents* or *ESAs*. They work by telling the body to make more red blood cells. Well-done studies have shown that they are able to reduce the need for getting blood transfusions in cancer patients treated with chemotherapy. A few good studies done outside the United States showed that giving an ESA to anemic prostate cancer patients on hormone therapy reduced their need for a blood transfusion and improved their quality-of-life.

Currently, ESAs are *not approved* in the United States for patients on hormone therapy. One reason is no good studies have proven if they are safe for men with this disease. Well-done studies in breast and lung cancer patients have shown ESAs can *shorten* survival, *increase* disease recurrence, and *increase* the risk of getting blood clots. Without further testing, your best advice at this time is to *not get an ESA* if you get anemic from hormone therapy. Given the increased safety of donated blood, blood transfusions are a better approach if you have symptoms from a low blood count. The use of an ESA is appropriate if you develop anemia while getting chemotherapy.

Weakness, decreased energy—Many men notice decreased energy, less ability to be active, and generalized weakness several months after starting hormone therapy. Well-done studies show that men who participate in a resistance exercise program had less interference from fatigue, had higher quality-of-life, and had higher levels of upper body and lower body muscular fitness than men not doing exercise. The program consisted of nine upper and lower strength-training exercises performed three times a week under the supervision of a fitness expert. Few doctors in the United States advise men to do any formal program, so you may have to seek out your own fitness trainer to set up a program for you.

Breast enlargement (gynecomastia)—All men have both testosterone and estrogen in their body. Normally, the ratio of estrogen to testosterone is low but that changes during hormone therapy resulting in breast enlargement. Only a small percentage of men are very bothered by it. In rare cases, plastic surgery is needed to reduce breast size. Giving two or three radiation treatments to the breast before starting hormone therapy can reduce the chance of it occurring. Some drugs also may be helpful. Tamoxifen (Nolvadex) is a hormonal drug used to treat breast cancer and it can reverse the gynecomastia. The FDA has not approved it for use in men. Even so, tamoxifen might be an option if you are severely bothered before you consider having surgery.

The Bottom Line About Hormone Therapy

Hormone therapy continues to be the best first-line treatment for metastatic prostate cancer despite the possible side effects. It can be done either by a short operation or using drugs placed under the skin. As more studies are done, another option may be to use estradiol applied to the skin. Intermittent hormone therapy could turn out to be a suitable alternative.

The good news is that continued discoveries have given you many more options making it possible to tailor the treatment for your specific needs and quality-of-life. Getting treated when you are first diagnosed with metastatic disease has more advantages over delayed therapy but it does cause side effects. You will have to weigh the choices and decide which approach you would prefer.

Managing Metastatic Disease With Combined Androgen Blockade or Triple Drug Therapy

What Are Antiandrogens?

In the previous chapter, the source of male hormones was described as mostly coming from the testicles with about 5% coming from the adrenal glands. Even the small amount from the adrenal glands can be enough to make prostate cancer cells grow. Another discovery made by Dr. Huggins was that some men with metastatic disease could benefit from removing both adrenal glands after castration was no longer working. The operation is called a *bilateral adrenalectomy*. Years later, doctors were able to make drugs called *antiandrogens* that have a similar effect on prostate cancer cells. They were discussed briefly in the previous chapter. The next table shows more details about the three antiandrogens approved by the FDA (Food and Drug Administration) to be taken in men with metastatic disease who will receive an LHRH drug.

Chemical Name	Flutamide	Bicalutamide	Nilutamide
Drug Name	Eulexin	Casodex	Nilandron
Dosing	two pills every eight hours	one pill per day	one pill per day
Most Common Side Effects	Breast tenderness and enlargement Liver changes Diarrhea	Breast tenderness and enlargement Liver changes	Breast tenderness and enlargement Liver changes Night Blindness Interstitial pneumonitis

Breast tenderness and gynecomastia—These side effects occur in approximately 33% to 67% of men on these drugs but few men are very bothered by them. Breast enlargement (gynecomastia) but not tenderness can be prevented using one to three doses of radiation delivered to the breasts before starting the drugs. Radiation is not effective after the breast enlargement has occurred. The dose of radiation needed has no side effects so you should strongly consider it if you are going to start one of these drugs. Studies are in progress to reverse gynecomastia, but the FDA has not yet approved any drug for that purpose.

Liver changes—All three antiandrogens can cause damage to the liver but only rarely is it life threatening. They should be used very cautiously in men with liver disease. In well-done studies, less than 1% of men had to stop the drug because of liver damage. If you take this drug, your liver function should be checked every few months by a blood test. If it becomes abnormal and does not get better in one or two months, then the antiandrogen should be stopped.

Diarrhea—This happens much more often in men taking flutamide compared to the other two drugs. In one well-done study, 24% of men getting flutamide had diarrhea compared to only 10% taking bicalutamide. When this happens for a man on flutamide, lowering the dose may help but its effectiveness against the cancer is not known. A safer approach is to switch to a different antiandrogen. The diarrhea will go away when the drug is stopped.

Night blindness—An unusual side effect of nilutamide is having difficulty driving at night when the light is low. It happens to about 12% to 14% of men taking this drug and the only treatment is to stop taking it.

Interstitial pneumonitis—This is an inflammation in the lung that results in fever, coughing, becoming short of breath, and having chest pain. It has been reported with all three antiandrogens but is about 10 times more common with nilutamide. For that reason, nilutamide should not be used in men with lung disease. The chances of this happening are about 17% in Japanese men but only 2% in other ethnic groups. Usually it goes away when the drug is stopped.

Which Antiandrogen Is Best for You?

The most commonly used antiandrogen in the United States is bicalutamide (Casodex). It may be the best first choice when one of these drugs is needed because of the following:

- It is taken only once per day.

- Less diarrhea occurs compared to flutamide.

- Night vision problems and interstitial pneumonia are avoided.

Bicalutamide is now a generic drug, which should drive down the price.

What Is Combined Androgen Blockade?

Years after Dr. Huggins' discovery of the benefit of removing the adrenal glands, some doctors asked the following question. Might patients do better by treating the adrenal hormones at the same time as doing medical or surgical castration? This treatment is called *combined androgen* blockade (CAB), maximum androgen blockade (MAB), complete androgen blockade or total androgen blockade (TAB). Despite more than 27 randomized studies having been done, doctors still disagree over the benefit and role of this treatment. The following are the most important results:

- Most studies were negative but three showed a much better survival with CAB compared to castration alone.

- At that time the studies were done, the longest average survival ever reported for men with metastatic prostate cancer getting CAB was 37 months. It was only 31 months in men getting castration alone.

- Men receiving CAB lived an average of three to six months longer than men getting castration alone followed by an antiandrogen given at a later time.

- In 2000, the results of all these studies were combined, showing that CAB resulted in a five-year survival rate of about 28% compared to 25% in men not getting CAB.

Despite these results, doctors still disagree about the value of CAB.

The Advantages and Disadvantages of Combined Androgen Blockade

Critics give four reasons why this treatment should not be given when you have metastatic prostate cancer. They are the following:

- Almost all the studies showed no benefit with CAB. If the treatment was really that good, then many more should have found a benefit.

- The increase in survival at five years was only 3%. That means 33 men have to be treated with CAB to help one man live longer.

- Increasing survival by an average of three to six months is not worth the added cost or the higher rate of side effects that occur with CAB.

- You can always get an antiandrogen later if the PSA begins to rise.

Doctors who favor CAB make the following arguments:

- Most of the studies did not enroll enough patients so they should be ignored.

- These studies were done before doctors knew that antiandrogens sometimes make the cancer worse. Studies done later showed that up to 50% of men improved when the drugs were stopped. This became known as the *antiandrogen withdrawal response (AAWR)*. It could explain why most studies did not show a benefit from CAB.

- Some studies suggested that CAB is most effective in men that don't have much metastatic disease. The studies may have been unsuccessful because most of the men in the studies had cancers that were very advanced.

- No study has shown that delaying the antiandrogen is as good as taking it immediately.

When Do You Stop the Antiandrogen?

Another disagreement among doctors is how long you should stay on CAB after starting it. Many prescribe the antiandrogen for only one month to prevent the flare response from a luteinizing hormone-releasing hormone (LHRH) agonist. Some doctors believe that using it longer may not be beneficial. They also do not recommend an antiandrogen when a man has surgical castration.

Other doctors believe that the only way to benefit from CAB is to use it until the PSA level begins to rise. They argue that no study has proven short-term use of CAB will help men live longer. One study suggested that men getting CAB for more than 120 days lived three times longer than men getting it for less time. If you want the best chance for increasing your survival, then take CAB until it is no longer effective.

How do doctors know when CAB is no longer helping you? The PSA is the best indicator. Many experts believe you should stop the antiandrogen when the PSA level goes up by 1 or 2 ng/mL on several tests, but there is no strict rule. You want to be sure it really is rising before stopping the drug. If the antiandrogen is stopped, you still should keep your testosterone level low because some cancer cells may grow faster when the level rises.

If your PSA level does rise and CAB is stopped, should another drug be started right away? The answer is no. You must first wait to see if you will get an antiandrogen withdrawal response. This will take one month if you have been using flutamide or nilutamide, but it could take two or even three months if you have been taking bicalutamide. During that time, be patient. If the PSA level does drop after stopping the antiandrogen, then you might not need any other treatment for four to six months.

What Is Triple Hormone Blockade?

Another treatment promoted by some doctors is called triple hormone blockade. It consists of combining CAB with a drug normally used to treat men who have symptoms from prostate enlargement. This third drug belongs to a group called 5-alpha-reductase inhibitors or 5-ARI drugs. They work by preventing normal prostate cells from converting testosterone to a more potent hormone called dihydrotestosterone or DHT. The FDA has approved two of them called finasteride (Proscar) and dutasteride (Avodart). They both improve urination and shrink the prostate.

Some doctors thought these drugs might also help men with prostate cancer because good studies show they prevent prostate cancer. Also, laboratory studies show these drugs stop cancer cells from growing in a plastic dish. One well-done study in men with metastatic disease found that taking 10 mg of finasteride a day for six weeks reduced the PSA by about 15%.

Is triple hormone therapy better than CAB? This question cannot be answered without a proper study. So far, no study has proven a true benefit. Nevertheless, some doctors and prostate cancer Web sites recommend triple androgen blockade as the *best* treatment for men with advanced disease.

Without proper studies, what should you do? Because finasteride and dutasteride have no major side effects, taking one of them with CAB is an option but don't be surprised if your doctor does not encourage it. As for those who strongly recommend them, you should be aware that it is only their personal opinion and it lacks good scientific proof. The bottom line is taking triple hormone therapy is an option, but you should understand that doctors do not know if it will help you.

The Bottom Line About Combined Androgen Blockade and Triple Hormone Therapy

Because more studies of CAB probably will never be done in the United States, the decision about its use must be made using the studies done many years ago. Although this combination may not cause a large increase in the average survival, it still is significant and some men may get a much greater benefit. CAB may not be for everyone, but you should at least discuss the pros and cons so you can make your own decision. That way, you can decide what is right for you. The bottom line is CAB is a good treatment if your goal is to do whatever you can to live as long as possible. In that case, do not wait until the cancer gets worse to add the antiandrogen because it appears to be less effective at that time. Doing it when metastatic disease is first detected is better than delaying it. If you choose to get CAB, then bicalutamide (Casodex) probably is the best one because it causes fewer side effects and can be taken once a day. If the PSA level rises, the first thing to do is to stop the antiandrogen and wait to see if the PSA improves. The testosterone level should continue to be kept low. At this time, the true value of triple drug therapy is unknown but it is an option. Hopefully, studies will be done to find out if it is a good thing to do.

Managing Androgen-Independent Prostate Cancer With Second-line Hormone Therapies

Although primary hormone therapy for metastatic disease will almost certainly help you for several years, its benefits usually do not often last forever. At some time, the cancer begins to progress. Doctors call this *androgen-independent prostate cancer (AIPC)*, *hormone refractory prostate cancer (HRPC)* or *castration-resistant prostate cancer (CRPC)*.

Do You Really Have Androgen-Independent Prostate Cancer?

Before you consider getting treated for AIPC, your doctor should check your testosterone level to be sure it is still less than the castrate level of 50 ng/mL. A higher level may make your cancer grow and reducing it may help you delay other treatments. As discussed in Chapter 25, the luteinizing hormone-releasing hormone (LHRH) agonists and the LHRH antagonist do not always keep the testosterone level under 50 ng/mL. If that happens to you, then the right treatment is either to switch to a different drug that lowers the testosterone level or have surgical castration. Your prostate-specific antigen (PSA) level then can be rechecked. No additional treatment is needed if it goes back down. If it still continues to rise, then another treatment may be appropriate.

Assuming your testosterone level is in the castrate range, your doctor has three ways to tell if you have AIPC:

- The PSA level increases.

- Your symptoms get worse.

- The bone scan or computerized axial tomography (CAT) scan shows new metastases or the existing ones get worse.

In almost every case, the PSA level will rise weeks or months before the symptoms or scans get worse. How much must the PSA level increase to say you have AIPC? There is no standard answer. Most doctors will not rely on just one increase, especially if it goes up by only a small amount. Some define AIPC as a percentage rise above the previous PSA level and others say it is three consecutive increases.

When Should You Consult an Oncologist?

Most men with advanced prostate cancer are treated by a urologist when they begin their initial hormone therapy. When AIPC develops, some urologists will make a referral to a medical oncologist whereas others will continue to do the treatment. The best time to start other therapies and the best option are not exactly known. Some doctors recommend chemotherapy when the PSA level begins to rise and others wait until symptoms develop. Because most urologists do not deliver chemotherapy, they often do not discuss it nor do they explain its pros and cons very well. That means you may not get fully informed about all your options. Getting a "second opinion" with an oncologist will help ensure you get all the information you need to make an informed decision about your next step. This has become even more important because more options are now available.

Options for Managing Androgen-Independent Prostate Cancer

The next question is, "How should you be treated when you have AIPC?" Your options include the following:

- Sit tight and do not get additional treatment until symptoms occur or the scans get worse.

- Begin *second-line hormone therapy*.

- Start *immunotherapy* or *chemotherapy*.

Arguments can be made for and against each choice. Although it sounds like a bad idea to do "nothing" when your PSA level is rising, delaying therapy allows you to avoid the side effects of other treatments. Although some treatments help you live longer, many men don't benefit. You may decide that the odds aren't great enough and you would prefer to wait. Fortunately, studies show you still can respond to chemotherapy even when it is delayed. Also, there is no proof that the results of chemotherapy are better if you are treated when the PSA level is 5 ng/mL, 10 ng/mL, 50 ng/mL, or even higher. Of course, if any of your symptoms are getting worse, then a "sit-tight" approach probably is not a good idea.

Many men with AIPC often make a "psychological decision" about when to get additional treatment. They are able to cope with a PSA level that remains under a certain number, but when it goes higher, they want something done. Each man has his own PSA level that will trigger a decision to get treated.

A second option for AIPC is called *second-line hormone therapy*. Some cancer cells still can respond to additional drugs that affect the male hormones. The reasons to use one of them are as follows:

- They lower the PSA level.

- They can reduce symptoms caused by the cancer.

- The side effects are usually milder and occur less often than those caused by chemotherapy drugs.

- Men still respond to chemotherapy and immunotherapy even if one or two second-line hormone therapies are used first.

The argument against using second-line hormone therapy is that doctors do not know if any of them improve survival because studies have not been done. Although it seems logical that lowering the PSA level and reducing symptoms *should* also improve survival, the fact is no one knows. This means the benefit of these drugs is more uncertain than the benefit of chemotherapy or immunotherapy. Also, most of them have not been approved by the FDA for treating progressive prostate cancer. Still, you may feel that the *package* of risks and benefits is more appealing than the other options and one of them may be appropriate for you.

The third option for AIPC is *chemotherapy*, which uses chemicals to kill cancer cells. The argument in favor of chemotherapy is it does improve survival. In 2004, the Food and Drug Administration (FDA) approved a drug called *docetaxel (Taxotere)* for the treatment of AIPC. Well-done studies showed that one half of the men getting this drug lived an *average* of two months longer than men not getting the drug or delaying it. Although two months may not seem like very much of a benefit, be aware that this is only an average. That means some men will have much more than a two-month increase in survival and others will have little or none. Because doctors cannot tell who will get a good response, the only way to have a chance of living longer is to try the drug. Chemotherapy may be most appropriate when you are having symptoms from your cancer. More details about this option is discussed in Chapter 29.

The last option is very new and it may totally change the approach to AIPC, at least for some men. In May 2010, the FDA approved *Provenge*, the very first *immunotherapy* for any type of cancer because studies showed it improved survival. One half of the men lived an average of about four months longer compared to the control group. This is a very exciting discovery because it gives doctors an entirely new type of treatment to offer men with AIPC. It works by stimulating a man's own immune system to fight the cancer. The details about Provenge are provided in Chapter 28.

Which Second-line Hormone Therapy Is Right for You?

Understanding the potential risks and benefits of each second-line hormone therapy will help you discuss the options with your doctor and decide if one of them is right for you. Studies have shown that 10% to 40% of men will respond to the drugs listed in the next table. In some cases, the PSA level doesn't go down but it does stop going up, which still may be helpful. The question is, "Which one is best for you?" At this time, no study has shown the best order for these drugs. Each has advantages and disadvantages and there is no "one size fits all." Until more studies are done, each doctor has his or her own personal approach. Fortunately, if you try one medication and it does not help or it helps and then stops working, you still may benefit from another one on the list. At any time, you can also consider switching to chemotherapy or immunotherapy.

Because there is no clear "best" approach, the treatment should be chosen based on your situation. You and your doctor should decide together which "package" is best for you. Although you should learn about all the options, don't be surprised if your doctor does not discuss some of them. This is another situation where you might benefit from a second opinion. The options are shown in the next table.

Second-line Hormonal Therapies

Options for Second-line Hormone Therapy	Major Side Effects	Frequency of Side Effects
Ketoconazole + hydrocortisone	Nausea	10%–30%
	Upset stomach	10%–30%
	Liver injury	Less than 0.1%
		All depend on dose used

Second-line Hormonal Therapies (Continued)

Options for Second-line Hormone Therapy	Major Side Effects	Frequency of Side Effects
Antiandrogens	All three drugs cause:	
A. Bicalutamide	Breast tenderness	60%–80%
(Casodex)	Breast enlargement and	60%–80%
B. Flutamide (Eulexin)	liver injury	Less than 0.01%
C. Nilutamide	Diarrhea (flutamide)	20%–24%
(Nilandron)	Difficulty with night vision (nilutamide)	13%–90%
	Interstitial pneumonia (nilutamide)	Less than 2%
Steroids	All three cause:	
A. Dexamethasone	Fluid retention	Frequency not reported
B. Prednisone	Diabetes	Frequency not reported
C. Hydrocortisone		
Estrogens	Fluid retention	17%–22%
A. Parenteral	Hypertension	18%–60%
—Polyestradiol	Breast enlargement	70%
phosphate (PEP)	Breast tenderness	42%
—Estradiol patch or gel		
B. Oral	Both oral drugs cause:	
—Diethylstilbestrol	Heart attacks	2%–5%
(DES)	Blood clots	2%–7%
—Estramustine	Breast tenderness	66%
(Emcyt)	Breast enlargement	7%
	Myocardial infarction	3%

Ketoconazole

This drug was approved many years ago by the FDA for the treatment of fungal infections but not for prostate cancer. Ketoconazole helps men with AIPC by blocking the production of male hormones in the adrenal gland. It may also directly kill prostate cancer cells. The daily dose ranges from 200 to 400 mg taken by mouth every eight hours. Doctors recommend taking it on an empty stomach because food decreases the absorption. Antacids should also be avoided within two hours of each dose. Most men tolerate the low and middle dose quite well but the higher dose may cause too much nausea. Doctors use three approaches to prescribing this drug.

- Option 1: Start with the lowest dose (200 mg every eight hours) and repeat the PSA test in one month. If the PSA level drops, then the same dose can be continued. If the PSA level does not change, then the dose can be increased. The PSA test should be repeated one month later to see if the higher dose has helped. If the PSA level still does not drop, then the drug should be stopped and a different treatment selected.

- Option 2: Start with the highest dose for one month and recheck the PSA level. If it declines without bothersome side effects occurring, then that dose is continued until the PSA level goes up. If this dose causes side effects, then it is reduced and the PSA level is checked again after one month. The drug should be discontinued if the PSA level does not go down.

- Option 3: Start with the middle dose (300 mg every eight hours). The PSA level is monitored monthly and if it begins to rise, then the higher dose can be tried for one month. If it goes up again, then the drug should be stopped.

This last option may make the most sense, but without good studies, they are all reasonable options. Although most men tolerate ketoconazole very well, about 10% to 30% will get an upset stomach. A potentially serious and life-threatening side effect is liver toxicity. Although it occurs in only 1 out of 10,000 individuals taking the drug, doctors are advised to do a blood test every few months to check the liver function.

This drug can also cause a drop in blood pressure in about 10% of patients. For that reason, many doctors prescribe a drug called *hydrocortisone* along with ketoconazole, which enables men to avoid this problem. This drug can also reduce cancer symptoms. The dose is 20 mg in the morning and 10 mg in the evening.

Antiandrogens

Antiandrogens were previously discussed in Chapter 26 as part of combined androgen blockade (CAB) and triple hormone therapy. Many doctors do not favor CAB when a man first develops metastatic disease. They prefer instead to delay giving the antiandrogen until the PSA level rises.

If you were on CAB and your PSA level increased, you still have about a 20% chance of responding to a different antiandrogen. Of course you must first stop the antiandrogen you are currently taking and wait to see if you get an antiandrogen withdrawal response. Only then is it appropriate to try a different antiandrogen.

If you have never received an antiandrogen, which one should you get first? The best choice probably is bicalutamide (Casodex) because of the following reasons:

- It is taken only once a day whereas flutamide (Eulexin) is taken three times per day.

- Flutamide causes diarrhea in more than 20% of men whereas it is very uncommon with bicalutamide.

- Nilutamide (Nilandron) can cause difficulty with night vision and interstitial pneumonia but neither one occurs with bicalutamide.

The dose of bicalutamide approved by the FDA for use with CAB is 50 mg per day. Some doctors recommend a dose of 150 mg a day (three tablets with a dose of 50 mg taken at the same time). Because there are no studies showing that the higher dose gives a better response and the drug can be costly, there is no good reason to take the higher amount. If that dose is ineffective, you probably are better off trying a different drug rather than taking more of it.

Suppose you already have taken bicalutamide and want to try a different antiandrogen, which one should be next? Both of them are reasonable because no studies have shown either is better. You can make the choice based on which of the possible side effects you find more acceptable. Diarrhea happens in about 20% to 24% of men on flutamide, and the problem with night vision occurs in up to 90% of men on nilutamide. If you must drive at night, then flutamide is obviously a better choice. If you are not driving at night, then nilutamide may be a better choice because it is only taken once per day and it does not cause diarrhea. Nilutamide is a better choice if you have loose bowel movements from previous radiation. Except for breast enlargement, the side effects will go away when you stop the drug. The dose of nilutamide is two 150 mg tablets per day taken at the same time for one month and then one pill a day thereafter. The FDA-approved dose of flutamide is two 125 mg tablets taken every eight hours. Some doctors use a lower dose to avoid the diarrhea but it is not known if it works as well.

Regardless of which drug you choose, try it for one month and then recheck the PSA level. If it has declined, then you can continue the drug. If the PSA level does not go down, then either try the other antiandrogen or change to a different treatment. Remember, you must wait at least four weeks after stopping an antiandrogen before trying a different treatment. Your liver function should be tested every two or three months because there is a 1% chance of liver toxicity with all three drugs.

Corticosteroids

Steroids are a group of chemicals produced in the body that control many body functions. *Corticosteroids* are steroids that are produced in the adrenal glands. Several synthetic corticosteroids have been developed that are used to treat inflammation. Although not specifically approved for prostate cancer, these drugs also lower the PSA level and reduce pain in men with AIPC. Corticosteroids are thought to work by reducing the male hormones produced in the adrenal glands.

The three corticosteroids used in men with prostate cancer are *prednisone*, *hydrocortisone*, and *dexamethasone*. They are all taken by mouth and are well tolerated. The medicine is best taken in the morning with some food to make it more tolerable and cause less stomach irritation. No studies have compared the three drugs to know if one is more effective. The doses that have been found to lower PSA levels are shown in the following table.

Doses of Corticosteroids

Drug	Dose
Prednisone	5–10 mg per day
Hydrocortisone	20–40 mg per day
Dexamethasone	0.75 mg 1–2 times per day

Prednisone and hydrocortisone have been used more often than dexamethasone for AIPC, which is the only reason to try those first. As with the other second-line hormone drugs, you try one and follow the PSA in one month. If your PSA level drops or remains stable, then it is reasonable to continue the drug. It should be stopped if the PSA level goes up. Most doctors will repeat the PSA test every month. It is unknown whether using a second corticosteroid is helpful after the initial one fails. Therefore, a better idea would be to try a different type of drug if your PSA level is increasing. The most common side effects of these medications include fluid retention called edema, increased blood pressure, and the development or worsening of diabetes.

If you do take a corticosteroid for several weeks, it is very important that you don't stop it abruptly, otherwise your blood pressure could suddenly drop. These drugs stop your adrenal gland from working properly, and it takes time for the gland to function normally again. Your daily dose is gradually reduced over five to seven days. Most, but not all, doctors know this, so don't hesitate to ask questions if you are told to stop a corticosteroid all at once.

Estrogens

When hormone therapy was first discovered in the 1940s, Dr. Huggins found that estrogen also helped men with advanced prostate cancer. A drug called diethylstilbestrol or DES initially was given by mouth at an initial dose of 5 mg per day. Unfortunately, this drug caused severe side effects. More men died from a heart attack or they developed blood clots. Although the dose was lowered, those side effects still can occur even at 1 mg per day. Some doctors recommend taking a blood thinner such as coumadin or aspirin to reduce the risk of blood clots. Another suggestion is to drink plenty of fluids to keep well hydrated. Neither treatment has been well studied.

Despite these risks, some doctors still recommend using 1 mg of DES per day. If you have a history of heart disease, it would be best not to use this drug without first getting approval from your cardiologist or family doctor. Because no studies show that DES is better than other second-line hormonal therapies, it would not be your best option. If you and your doctor decide to use it, the PSA should be monitored every one or two months. The drug can be continued if you tolerate it well and the PSA level declines. Switching to a different drug is a safer choice than raising the dose.

Fortunately, when estrogens are given parenterally, these complications are much less common. Parenteral routes for this drug include placing a patch or gel on the skin or injecting them into a vein, a muscle, or under the skin.

Another estrogen approved by the FDA is called estramustine (Emcyt). It is taken by mouth at a dose based on each man's weight. It has almost the same frequency of side effects as 3 mg of DES. Few doctors choose it for AIPC because better choices are available.

Both parenteral and oral estrogens do have one advantage over other second-line hormonal therapies. They can potentially protect against osteoporosis that occur more often in men getting surgical castration or an LHRH drug. They also can lower cholesterol. Studies are needed to determine if parenteral estrogens truly are safer. Currently, the FDA has not approved them for men with prostate cancer but some doctors use them anyway.

If you decide to be treated with parenteral estrogen, which route is best for you? Placing patches on your skin may be easiest and more convenient than receiving an injection every two weeks. Each patch contains 0.1 mg of *estradiol*. It is usually placed on the abdomen and changed approximately every three to four days. The location of the patches does not appear to influence how well they work. Studies are in progress to determine the proper dosing that will keep the testosterone level below 50 ng/dL. Weak studies found a drop in the PSA level from using two patches changed every three or four days. That seems like a reasonable approach until results of ongoing studies become available. The PSA can be measured after one month and the symptoms can be assessed before deciding what to do. This dose can be continued if your PSA level declines and/or you feel better. If neither occurs, then the dose can be increased to three or four patches twice a week or a different treatment can be tried. Following your testosterone levels is not very helpful because it should already be less than 50 ng/dL. More information is needed to know the proper dosing of estradiol gel.

The other parenteral estrogen is an intramuscular injection of *polyestradiol phosphate* (PEP). Good studies have compared this drug to an LHRH agonist in men getting primary hormone therapy for advanced prostate cancer. The results showed a similar survival. The dose used was 240 mg injected into the muscle every two weeks for two months followed by 240 mg every month. This dosing schedule was able to lower testosterone to a castrate level as often as an LHRH medication when given as "first-line" treatment.

No studies have been done using PEP as a second-line treatment. Until studies become available, the best advice is to use the same dosing schedule for second-line therapy as was used for primary therapy. The PSA should be checked after one month and the medication can be continued until the PSA level increases.

What Happens to My Primary Hormone Therapy When I Start a New Treatment?

What should you do about your LHRH drug when starting a second-line hormonal drug? Should you stop it because it is no longer controlling the cancer or does it still help you in some way? Although no good studies have been done, most experts recommend you continue to keep your testosterone level less than 50 ng/dL. They believe the cancer will grow faster if the testosterone level is allowed to rise.

Some doctors suggest a different approach. Studies have shown that sometimes the testosterone will stay low even after stopping the LHRH drug. The testicles seem to lose their ability to make testosterone. For that reason, the drug can be stopped and the testosterone rechecked. No further treatment is needed if the testosterone stays low. The main advantages of doing this are comfort, convenience, and cost because injections would no longer be necessary. The one downside is if the testosterone level rises and an LHRH agonist is restarted. A new "flare response" might occur during the first injection, although drugs may prevent it.

The Bottom Line About Second-line Hormone Therapies

Doctors are still not sure whether any second-line hormone therapy helps men live longer. They do seem to reduce cancer symptoms and lower the PSA level in approximately 10% to 40% of men. The good news is that some men respond for more than a year. Those benefitting are able to avoid going on other treatments. Because no one can predict if you will benefit, all risks and benefits of all second-line agents should be discussed as options for treating your androgen-independent prostate cancer. That way you can help decide what to do.

Immunotherapy Using Sipuleucel-T

What Is Your Immune System?

The immune system is your body's defense against things that may harm you such as bacteria, viruses, wounds, and even cancer. It is a complicated interaction between certain organs, cells, and chemicals made by your body. These work together when threatened by something "foreign." Your immune system is much better at defending against germs than cancer cells. Germs are very clearly foreign but cancer cells have some things in common with normal cells in your body. Cancer cells also release certain chemicals that protect them from being destroyed by the body. Using the immune system to fight disease is called immunotherapy.

How Does Your Immune System Work?

Any substance your body thinks is foreign can stimulate an immune response. These foreign substances are called antigens. Usually they are present on the surface of invading cells. When an antigen enters the body, several types of normal cells work together in a complicated way to kill the foreign cells directly or help the body get rid of them. One type is called a dendritic cell. These cells are very effective but not many of them are normally in the body.

For years, doctors have searched for ways to improve the ability of the immune system to fight cancer cells with little success. That all changed when studies showed that the survival of men with advanced prostate cancer could be improved by a treatment named *sipuleucel-T*.

What Is Sipuleucel-T and How Is the Treatment Done?

This is a vaccine therapy that stimulates the body's own immune system. The treatment involves several steps that include the following:

- Collecting your blood and separating the dendritic cells and other lymphocytes by a process called *leukapheresis*.

- Combining these cells with *prostatic acid phosphatase* for about 40 hours. It is an antigen located on the surface of most prostate cancer cells. This produces "activated" cells called sipuleucel-T.

- These activated cells are given back to you three days later into a vein. They stimulate other normal cells to kill the prostate cancer in your body.

- The process is repeated two more times over about four weeks.

What Are the Results With Sipuleucel-T?

Considerable controversy has surrounded this treatment. The initial two studies were designed to determine if sipuleucel-T would delay progression of the cancer in men with metastatic disease. Neither of them accomplished that goal but additional follow-up showed that men receiving sipuleucel-T lived longer than men in the control group. Despite this result, the Food and Drug Administration (FDA) did not approve the treatment and instead required that another study be done.

In the next study, more than 500 men with androgen-independent prostate cancer (AIPC) received either sipuleucel-T or cells that were not exposed to the prostatic acid phosphatase. The results showed that one half of the men getting sipuleucel-T lived about 4.1 months longer than the men in the control group. At 36 months, 32% of the men receiving sipuleucel-T were still alive compared to only 23% of men in the control group. Based on this result, the FDA approved this treatment in April 2010. The treatment has been named *Provenge*.

What Are the Side Effects of Sipuleucel-T?

Almost everyone in the randomized studies reported having some side effects as shown in the following table.

Frequency of Side Effects in Randomized Study

Side Effects	Sipuleucel-T Group	Control Group
Chills	53%	11%
Fatigue	41%	35%
Fever	31%	10%
Back pain	30%	29%
Nausea	22%	15%
Joint ache	20%	21%
Headache	18%	7%
Vomiting	13%	8%

Frequency of Side Effects in Randomized Study (Continued)

Side Effects	Sipuleucel-T Group	Control Group
Pain	12%	7%
Muscle ache	12%	6%
Weakness	11%	7%
Diarrhea	10%	11%
Flulike illness	10%	4%
Musculoskeletal pain	9%	10%
Shortness of breath	9%	5%
Hypertension	8%	5%
Sweating	5%	1%

These side effects need little explanation. Fortunately, few of them were very serious. Chills, fatigue, and fever were most common. You may wonder why so many side effects occurred in the control group. One reason is that the cancer may have caused some of them. Another possibility is because blood cells were removed from the body, kept in a laboratory for 40 hours, and then given back to those men three days later.

How severe were some of these side effects? When clinical studies are done, side effects are graded on a scale of 1 to 5. For this study, the following descriptions were used:

- Grade 1 = Mild side effects

- Grade 2 = Moderate side effects

- Grade 3 = Severe side effects

- Grade 4 = Life-threatening or disabling side effects
- Grade 5 = Fatal side effects

Mild and moderate side effects are not serious and do not require much treatment. Treatments are needed when side effects are severe or life threatening. The study found about 25% of the men had severe side effects but in only 4% were they were life threatening.

Who Is a Candidate for Sipuleucel-T?

The study was specifically designed to treat men with AIPC who had few, if any, symptoms from their cancer. For that reason, only those men are eligible to get treated at this time. One problem is that the treatment may be in short supply until later in 2011 when more processing plants become available. Also, only select doctors will be allowed to give this treatment, which may change in the future.

For now, men with AIPC may prefer to have sipuleucel-T before considering chemotherapy. Although both cause side effects, they are more serious with docetaxel. Also, this immunotherapy requires only three treatments but chemotherapy must be given every three weeks. If you are interested in this treatment and your doctor does not use it, you can visit the company Web site to find a physician near you who can give it (www.provenge.com).

The treatment will be quite expensive. Initial estimates are that the three injections will cost between $90,000 and $100,000. Several insurance companies and Medicare have already approved paying for it, although in June 2010, Medicare has decided to conduct a lengthy review about covering it.

The Bottom Line About Sipuleucel-T

The approval of Provenge is a major advance in treating prostate cancer and is likely to result in studies testing it earlier in the disease. Spending nearly $100,000 for about four extra months of survival may seem overly expensive but is in line with other cancer therapies. The good news is that it is yet another treatment that can help improve survival if you have progressed during hormone therapy. Although side effects may be common, they are less serious compared to chemotherapy. For that reason, you may decide to do it first and then receive docetaxel if it isn't helping. You still can respond to chemotherapy later.

If you do get sipuleucel-T, be aware that your PSA and your bone scan will not be good indicators of whether you are responding. Neither one improved during the study even though men getting the treatment lived longer. This will create some problem in deciding whether the Provenge is not working and you should get a different treatment. The bottom line is sipuleucel-T is an important advance in the treatment of advanced prostate cancer.

Chemotherapy

29

Chemotherapy is a broad term that means using chemicals to treat a disease. *Cytotoxic chemotherapy* uses drugs that kill cells. Many cytotoxic chemotherapy drugs have been discovered over the years to treat cancer. Several have been approved to treat prostate cancer. Chemotherapy is not used initially for metastatic prostate cancer because the tumor responds well to hormone therapy. It is mainly used when hormone therapy is no longer controlling the disease. The terms for it are *androgen-independent prostate cancer (AIPC), castration-resistant prostate cancer (CRPC)* or *hormone-resistant prostate cancer (HRPC).* Details about AIPC were explained in detail in Chapter 27. Important facts you may not know about cytotoxic chemotherapy drugs are the following:

- Some cancers respond very well to certain drugs but are totally unaffected by others.

- Normal cells are also affected, which can lead to serious side effects.

- These drugs rarely kill all the cancer cells in a person's body. Some cells are resistant or become resistant and they can continue to grow.

Since 1999, the Food and Drug Administration (FDA) has approved three chemotherapy drugs for men with AIPC. The chemical and trade names are:

- mitoxantrone (Novantrone)

- docetaxel (Taxotere)

- carbazitaxel (Jevtana)

Mitoxantrone (Novantrone)

This chemotherapy drug was approved for treating men with prostate cancer based on well-done studies showing it could palliate or reduce pain caused by the disease. It also lowered the use of pain medication and improved quality-of-life but it did not prolong survival. The drug is given every three weeks through a vein over 30 minutes. Mitoxantrone usually is combined with 5 mg of prednisone given two times each day.

How much does it help patients? In one of three good studies, men were assigned to get mitoxantrone plus prednisone or prednisone alone. Patients completed written surveys that asked about their quality-of-life and their use of drugs to treat pain. Quality-of-life improved in about 30% of the men getting the two drugs compared to only 12% in men getting prednisone alone. One half of the men in the mitoxantrone group responded for about 7.6 months compared to only 2.1 months in the control group. The men in the control group eventually could receive mitoxantrone after six weeks if their symptoms got worse. About 20% of those men responded. This suggests the drug may be slightly more effective when used sooner rather than later.

The following table shows a comparison of the important side effects occurring in this study followed by an explanation of the medical terms. They were far more common in the group getting mitoxantrone.

Side Effects of Mitoxantrone

Side Effect	Mitoxantrone + Prednisone	Prednisone Alone
Neutropenia	87%	4%
Anemia	75%	39%
Nausea	26%	8%
Fatigue	34%	14%
Alopecia	22%	1%
Anorexia	22%	14%
Infections	17%	4%
Edema	10%	4%
Stomatitis	8%	1%
Vomiting	11%	5%
Night sweats	9%	2%
Hematuria	11%	6%
Dyspnea	15%	8%

Neutropenia—a decrease in the number of white blood cells in the body, which increases the risk for developing infections.

Anemia—a decrease in the number of red blood cells in the body. Red blood cells deliver oxygen to the body. When the number of red blood cells drops, men may feel weak, tired, and short of breath during exertion. Advanced prostate cancer often causes anemia and mitoxantrone may make it worse. Blood transfusions are needed if the red blood cells drop very low. Another option is to give drugs that help the body make more red blood cells.

Alopecia—means loss of hair, either on the head or all over the body. Many chemotherapy drugs cause hair loss, which usually grows back if the drug is stopped.

Stomatitis—inflammation in the mouth that can lead to open sores. It may be very bothersome because chewing is painful and some foods or liquids can be quite irritating.

Hematuria—This is the term for the appearance of red blood cells in the urine. Depending on the amount, it can turn the urine red. Rarely, blood clots appear in the urine. Treatment is unnecessary unless a clot blocks the urine.

Dyspnea—difficulty catching your breath or feeling short of breath during physical exertion.

The Bottom Line About Mitoxantrone

When you read the long list of side effects, your first thought might be, "Why would I ever consider taking this drug?" Keep in mind that despite all of them, men taking the drug still felt it improved their quality-of-life and reduced their use of pain medication. The trade-off seemed worthwhile to those men. Clearly, if your pain from the cancer is only mild, then this drug probably is not for you. But if you require narcotics or you have trouble moving or sleeping, then the benefits of the drug outweigh its side effects. Now that three other treatments are available that improve survival, mitoxantrone probably should be delayed until the other therapies no longer help you.

Docetaxel (Taxotere)

Docetaxel belongs to a group of drugs called *taxanes* that come from yew trees. In 2004, two good studies showed that *docetaxel* could improve survival in men with AIPC. Based on those studies, the FDA approved this drug. It is given intravenously (through a vein) over about one hour.

In one study, men with AIPC were assigned to one of three groups. One was given docetaxel and prednisone weekly, the second group was given the two drugs every three weeks, and the control group was given mitoxantrone and prednisone every three weeks. The study found that the group getting the docetaxel and prednisone every three weeks had a significantly better survival than men getting mitoxantrone and prednisone. One half of the men survived about 18.9 months compared to only 16.9 months for the control group. That means one half of the men getting docetaxel lived about two months longer than the men getting mitoxantrone. They were also more likely to have their pain reduced, which occurred in 35% compared to only 20% in the control group. This means about one out of every six men felt better while taking the drug. Weekly docetaxel was no better than mitoxantrone. The frequency of side effects is shown in the next table followed by an explanation of some of the terms.

Side Effects of Docetaxel

Side Effects	Docetaxel + Prednisone Every Three Weeks	Mitoxantrone + Prednisone Every Three Weeks
Anemia	5%	2%
Neutropenia	32%	22%
Worsening heart function	10%	22%
Fatigue	53%	35%
Alopecia	65%	13%
Nail changes	30%	7%

Side Effects of Docetaxel (Continued)

Side Effects	Docetaxel + Prednisone Every Three Weeks	Mitoxantrone + Prednisone Every Three Weeks
Nausea, vomiting	42%	38%
Diarrhea	32%	10%
Neuropathy	30%	7%
Anorexia	17%	14%
Dysgeusia	18%	7%
Stomatitis	20%	8%
Myalgia	14%	13%
Dyspnea	15%	9%
Tearing	10%	1%
Peripheral edema	19%	1%
More than one serious event	26%	20%

Neutropenia—a decrease in the number of white blood cells in the body, which increases the risk for developing infections.

Nail changes—includes a change in the color of the nail bed, or the nail breaks easily.

Neuropathy—a feeling of burning or tingling in the fingers and toes.

Dysgeusia—a change in the taste of food.

Myalgia—pain in the muscles.

Tearing—the eyes easily water.

Edema—collection of fluid in the body usually occurring in the lower part of the legs.

Despite the higher incidence of side effects in men getting docetaxel, they still had a better overall quality-of-life. Also, their frequency of serious side effects was only 6% higher compared to the control group.

The second good study combined docetaxel with another che-motherapy drug called *estramustine* (Emcyt). These two were compared to mitoxantrone and prednisone. The docetaxel and the mitoxan-trone were given intravenously every three weeks. Estramustine is an estrogen-containing pill that was approved many years ago for men with advanced prostate cancer. It is now used infrequently because of its side effects.

This study also found that men getting docetaxel and estramustine lived longer than those getting mitoxantrone and prednisone. One half of the men survived 17.5 months compared to only 15.6 months in the control group, a difference of about two months. Another advantage was the time it took for the cancer to get worse. It was 6.3 months in the docetaxel group but only 3.2 months in the control group. Side effects were common, but some probably were caused by the estramustine.

The Bottom Line About Docetaxel

Although the improvement in survival is not very large, it still represents a significant advance in the treatment of AIPC. The best time to get this drug is unclear. Should it be started when the PSA level begins to rise during hormone therapy or not until the disease is causing symptoms? This becomes another choice between sur-vival and quality-of-life. The drug can help you live longer but may cause bothersome side effects. Is the trade-off worth it? Only you can decide. If you are not having any symptoms when your PSA level is rising and you feel well, delaying treatment may be best. Fortunately, docetaxel still can help when used later in the disease.

Carbazitaxel (Jevtana)

In June 2010, the FDA approved *carbazitaxel (Jevtana)* for men with AIPC. The drug has a chemical structure similar to docetaxel and it is also given through a vein over one hour. It was tested in men that progressed while receiving docetaxel. They were assigned to receive either prednisone and mitoxantrone (the control group) or prednisone and carbazitaxel every month for up to 10 months. Men getting carbazitaxel and prednisone lived longer than men in the control group. One half of them were alive at 15.1 months compared to only 12.7 months in those getting mitoxantrone and prednisone.

The trade-off with this drug is the type, frequency, and severity of the side effects. About 1 out of 20 men (5%) died from getting carbazitaxel. This partly occurred because medications that would have protected most men were not allowed during the first month. Therefore, anyone now starting carbazitaxel is advised to take drugs that reduce the risk of a life-threatening side effect. Another caution is that the drug can cause severe allergic reactions. The frequency of the most common and significant side effects occurring during this study is shown in the next table. Grade 1 (mild) and grade 2 (moderate) side effects are somewhat annoying and bothersome but not dangerous, grade 3 (severe) and grade 4 (life threatening) are much more dangerous. The side effects not described earlier are explained in the following table.

Side Effects of Carbazitaxel

Side Effects in Men Receiving Carbazitaxel + Prednisone	Grade 1 or 2	Grade 3 or 4	Total Having Side Effect
Leukopenia	27%	69%	96%
Anemia	87%	11%	98%
Thrombocytopenia	44%	4%	48%
Neutropenia	12%	82%	94%

Side Effects of Carbazitaxel (Continued)

Side Effects in Men Receiving Carbazitaxel + Prednisone	Grade 1 or 2	Grade 3 or 4	Total Having Side Effect
Nausea	32%	2%	34%
Vomiting	20%	2%	22%
Diarrhea	41%	6%	47%
Constipation	19%	1%	20%
Abdominal pain	15%	2%	17%
Fatigue	32%	5%	37%
Pyrexia	11%	1%	12%
Asthenia	15%	5%	20%
Urinary tract infection	6%	2%	8%
Anorexia	15%	1%	16%
Back pain	12%	4%	16%
Peripheral neuropathy	12%	1%	13%
Dysgeusia	11%	0%	11%
Hematuria	15%	2%	17%
Dysuria	7%	0%	7%
Alopecia	10%	0%	10%
Dyspnea	11%	1%	12%

Leukopenia—a drop in the number of white blood cells in the blood stream, which increases the chances of developing infections.

Thrombocytopenia—a drop in the number of platelets in the blood stream, which increases the chances of bleeding.

Pyrexia—the development of a fever.

Asthenia—muscle weakness.

Peripheral neuropathy—a feeling of burning or tingling in the fingers and toes.

Dysuria—burning or pain during urination.

The Bottom Line About Carbazitaxel

Until this drug was approved, men getting worse while on docetaxel had few or no other good options. They could get pain relief from mitoxantrone but that drug did not help increase survival. This clearly is an important advance but it also has significant risks. Good oncologists will monitor you carefully when you receive this drug and give you other drugs to reduce your risk of getting some of the side effects. Although you might also be very reluctant to take this medication, remember to look at the whole "package" of risks and benefits. Some men may get a greater increase in survival than others. Doctors are working on ways to tell which patient is more likely to benefit. If the cancer is progressing, your hope of prolonging your survival will require you to accept more risks. If, however, you are more concerned about your quality-of-life at this stage of your disease, then other drugs are available that can reduce your symptoms. In that case, carbazitaxel may not be the right thing for you to do.

Treatment Options for Bone Metastases

When prostate cancer spreads into the bones, it can cause pain and fractures. In rare cases, it may even cause a spinal cord compression leading to paralysis. The net result is a worsening of a man's quality-of-life. Fortunately, improvements in treatment have made these events less common.

How Are Bone Metastases Monitored?

The bone scan continues to be the most sensitive way to detect or monitor bone metastases. You already have had a bone scan showing cancer in the bones. Another one will be done if your prostate-specific antigen (PSA) level continues to rise. Doctors use different PSA levels to make this decision. There is not a "best" approach. If you get new bone pain, the scan will be repeated regardless of your PSA level. Repeat scans will be done every several months as needed.

After a bone scan is performed, it is compared to the previous one to see if new "spots" have appeared or previous spots have gotten worse. Your doctor should determine if cancer has spread into your weight-bearing bones like the hip, femur, or spine. In those cases, plain X-rays, a computed axial tomography (CAT) scan, or magnetic resonance imaging (MRI) scan of those bones are recommended. The goal is to see if a fracture has occurred or a bone is at risk for fracturing in the near future. These tests are necessary because not all the spots seen on a bone scan are caused by metastases. They could be caused by a healed fracture, arthritis, or other noncancerous conditions. Rarely, a biopsy of a bone must be performed to find out why the scan is abnormal. If your PSA level is rising and new spots are seen, most likely it means your cancer has gotten worse. After confirming that a weight-bearing bone could fracture or if you have bone pain, the next step is to arrange for a consultation with a radiation therapist.

What Are the Options for Treating Bone Metastases?

In addition to taking drugs to relieve the pain, several bone-specific treatments can also be given including the following:

- external radiation

- radiopharmaceuticals (radioactive isotopes)

- bisphosphonates

External Radiation for Bone Metastases

Some doctors use the term *spot radiation* when one or involved bones is given this treatment. The same machines are used to treat bone metastases as are used for treating the prostate. The difference is the bones respond to a much smaller amount of radiation. Good studies have shown that *a single treatment is as effective as 30 of them.* You may be surprised to learn that the number of treatments and total dose given to the bones is quite variable throughout the United States. A large survey found that about one half of the radiotherapists give 10 treatments. If you are going to receive this treatment for your pain and are told it will take one to two weeks, ask, "Why is more than one dose needed when there is no proof it is better?" More radiation will be given if a bone has been very damaged.

About one fourth of men get complete relief of pain from spot radiation. Another 41% can expect more than one half of their pain to decrease within one month of being radiated. Usually, it is well tolerated and causes almost no side effects.

Radiopharmaceuticals (Radioisotopes)

Radiopharmaceuticals are drugs that contain a radioactive compound. When injected into a vein, they circulate throughout the body, find their way into bones invaded by cancer, and then give off their radiation. They can kill cancer cells and relieve pain or protect the bone from fracturing in the future. The radiation only extends a short distance away from the radioactive material so the whole body is not affected. Small amounts do stay in some normal parts of the body. They include the bone marrow and the wall of the colon, bladder, testicles, and kidneys.

The most common side effects are a lowering of the white blood cells and platelets. For that reason, frequent blood tests are done to monitor the blood counts especially when you are also getting chemotherapy. Blood products may be needed if the cell counts drop too low.

Eventually, the radiation goes away or decays depending on its half-life, which is the time required for one half of the radiation to disappear. The amount of the radiopharmaceutical given will depend on your weight. Most of the radioactivity gets out of the body through the urine. Although men are advised to make sure all the urine is emptied into the toilet bowl, a few drops of urine "missing the mark" is unlikely to harm anyone.

Strontium-89 (^{89}Sr) (Metastron)

This radioisotope has been used for bone metastases for more than 15 years. It has a half-life of 55 days in bones containing cancer but only 14 days in normal bones. That means the radiation is almost completely gone from you body in about eight months. Your pain usually will be improved within one to three weeks after the injection. Older studies showed that about 65% of men receiving ^{89}Sr plus external radiation had a significant drop in bone pain in six months compared to only 35% receiving external radiation alone. Blood counts drop in two to four weeks and gradually return to their baseline level over the next 12 weeks. At that time, another dose can be given if needed.

Samarium-153 (^{153}Sm) (Quadramet)

This agent has a half-life of only 46 hours so the radiation will disappear from your body much faster than with ^{89}Sr. It also is excreted in the urine so the same precautions should be used. You should drink plenty of fluids and urinate often to minimize the amount of radiation affecting your bladder. Studies show that by three weeks, 53% of patients getting ^{153}Sm had significant improvement in pain compared to 25% of men getting a placebo. The treated group also was able to reduce their intake of narcotics.

^{153}Sm caused about a 50% drop in white blood cell counts and platelets but serious complications occurred in very few patients. If you get this treatment, your blood counts should be measured every two weeks. No studies have been done to find out if ^{153}Sm is better than ^{89}Sr so both are reasonable choices. ^{153}Sm has the advantage of disappearing from your body more quickly.

Doctors have different opinions about whether to use spot radiation or one of these radiopharmaceuticals. Spot radiation may be safer and more convenient if only a few bones are treated but it may cause more permanent damage to the bone marrow if multiple bones need treatment. In that case, a radiopharmaceutical is a better choice. Sometimes both are used.

Bisphosphonates

A two-step process called remodeling is constantly renewing the bones in our body. In the first step, old bone is broken down and removed, and in the second step, new bone is formed. Prostate cancer that has spread to the bones can interfere with this remodeling. *Bisphosphonates* work by stopping the breakdown of bones, which makes them useful when you have bone metastases or osteoporosis.

In one study done in men on hormone therapy who had metastatic disease and a rising PSA level, one group was assigned to get a bisphosphonate called *zoledronic acid (Zometa)* and the other group received a placebo. The drugs were given intravenously every three weeks for 15 months. Zoledronic acid was tested at two doses: 4 and 8 mg. The goal of the study was to compare quality-of-life, pain, and the frequency of *skeletal-related events* (SRE), which included the following:

- bone fractures caused by prostate cancer

- compression of the spinal cord

- radiation treatment to involved bones

- surgery on a bone affected by the cancer

- a change of therapy because of worsening cancer

The key results are shown in the next table.

Result	Zoledronic Acid 4 mg	Placebo
SRE	38%	49%
Fracture due to cancer	13%	22%
Median time to first SRE	488 days	321 days

The study showed a significant benefit from the 4-mg dose of the drug. For every nine men getting treated, one avoided getting a skeletal-related event. Also, one-half of the men getting zoledronic acid developed their first SRE 167 days later than half of the group getting the placebo. Pain scores and quality-of-life measurements did not differ at 15 months. Based on this study, the Food and Drug Administration (FDA) approved the drug for men with bone metastases who were getting worse during hormone therapy.

The drug did not cause many significant side effects as shown in the next table.

Side Effect	Zoledronic Acid	Placebo
Fatigue	33%	26%
Anemia	27%	18%
Decreased kidney function	15%	12%

Doctors have learned that the problems occurring with kidney function are partly due to how fast the drug is given. Now, the safest approach is to make sure the drug is delivered no faster than 15 minutes. Also, kidney function should be measured by a simple blood test before each treatment. If your kidney function is not normal, then the dose should be reduced or the treatment delayed until the kidneys improve.

Since the study was done, another complication was discovered that occurs with any bisphosphonate. It is called *osteonecrosis of the jaw* or ONJ. It is defined as the development of pain, swelling, and decreased healing following a dental procedure such as removing a tooth. ONJ is more common in men getting intravenous treatment compared to taking a bisphosphonate by mouth. Also, the longer the drug is used, the greater is the chance that ONJ will occur. One study found it developed in about 1% of men after 12 months, 7% after 24 months, and 21% after four years of taking zoledronic acid. For that reason, you are advised to have good dental care. If you need oral surgery, make sure your dentist knows you are taking this drug.

The Bottom Line About Zoledronic Acid

This drug is another good example of the importance of weighing risks and benefits. Zoledronic acid does help a small number of men who have cancer in the bones. Most of the benefit is avoiding radiation to the bones in the future but overall quality-of-life is not improved. The question for you to decide is whether getting a drug intravenously every three weeks is worth the risks. The good news is that several good options exist to help when you have problems from bone metastases.

Summary of Managing Bone Metastases

Bone metastases from prostate cancer can have severe consequences. Fortunately, good options are available to reduce the chances that they will occur and others may soon become available. One of them is denosumab (Chapter 32) which has completed clinical testing and showed a greater benefit than zoledronic acid. The FDA is expected to make their decision regarding approval in the very near future. This is an important part of managing your disease so make sure to discuss these options with your doctor.

Is a Research Study Right for You?

31

A clinical research study is actually an experiment done on individuals to determine if a test or a treatment is safe and effective. Progress in treating prostate cancer can only occur if research studies or trials are done, which requires that men must be willing to volunteer. These studies can be designed in different ways called *phases*. Each has different goals and different rules.

A *phase I* study is done when laboratory studies suggest that a new treatment *may* help individuals with a specific illness. Initially, little is known about how to give it, when to give it, how much to use and whether it is safe or effective. In a phase I study, everyone is given the experimental treatment but the dose and timing will vary. At the end of this study, a dose, frequency, and method of giving the drug will be selected for use in a *phase II* study. Participating in a phase I study makes the most sense for people who have few other options for treating their illness. Although there is no proof it will work, some men *might* get a very good response. It is the only way to get this treatment without having to wait many years until it is readily available.

A *phase II* study is done to test if a treatment is able to improve individuals who have a particular disease. The goal is to search for some evidence that patients are responding such as reducing symptoms or improving a blood test or X-ray. In a phase II study, everyone gets the experimental treatment but some people may get a smaller amount that is not expected to be effective. Potential side effects are recorded. The results of a phase II study will be used to determine whether the treatment should be taken into the next study phase. A phase II study is also used to identify which individuals are best suited for the next evaluation.

The *phase* III study is the most important one because the Food and Drug Administration (FDA) uses the results to decide if a drug is safe and effective and should be approved for patient care. These studies must be prospective, randomized, and controlled. This means only some people are *assigned* to get the experimental treatment. Others get the "standard" treatment used for treating that disease at the time the study is set to begin. *In a phase III study, participants cannot choose their therapy.*

The final study design is called a *phase IV* trial. It is done after the FDA has already approved that treatment. The goal is to learn more about its longer-term risks, side effects, and benefits. It will include many more individuals than the phase III study.

Should You Join a Research Study?

Nothing is wrong with feeling reluctant to sign up for a research study. After all, it may seem like you would be a "guinea pig" and you are concerned about your safety. Fortunately, strict guidelines exist in the United States and many other countries that regulate how research studies are performed. They require protection of everyone joining a study and following good clinical practice. That protection includes an individual's rights, welfare, and safety. The rules do vary slightly for studies testing drugs as compared to medical devices. Another way individuals are protected is by having all clinical research studies reviewed and approved by a hospital or university before they can begin. Also, physicians who conduct research on new drugs are monitored to ensure they are complying with the rules governing research.

Perhaps, you may not want to enroll because many studies require that the treatments be randomized. This means neither you nor your doctor have any control in deciding whether you get the "standard" or "experimental" treatment. You must understand that the only way to find out if one treatment is as good, better, or worse than another one is to test it in a randomized study.

Two points that may make you less reluctant to sign up for a phase III study are:

- You will never be deprived of a treatment that has been proven to help men in your situation. If something has been shown to be beneficial, you can expect that everyone in the study will get it as part of the "control" group. Some of the participants will also get the "experimental" treatment.

- If you are randomized to the control group, you are no worse off than if you never joined the study because you are getting the same treatment you would normally receive.

The Benefits and Risks of Enrolling in a Research Study

Joining a research study has several benefits that include the following:

- You get a chance to receive a promising new treatment many years before it will be available to the general public. That is the only way to get that treatment without having to wait several years until it is "approved." This may be most important if you already have tried all the conventional treatments and your disease is getting worse. Perhaps your disease has a high risk of recurring and you want to try something to improve your odds of surviving.

- You will be more closely monitored with tests and exams than if you just received routine care.

- You get the satisfaction of knowing you may be helping others by contributing to medical research.

- If you do not have good health insurance, you may be able to get access to doctors and treatments that would not be possible without enrolling.

- Some studies will pay you money to participate.

Of course, there also are the following potential risks:

- You might get side effects from the experimental treatment. Before enrolling, you will be told what ones are known but doctors may not be aware of all of them. They also will not know exactly how often they occur until the study has been completed.

- The study could be time consuming, requiring you to undergo extra tests or see a doctor more often than if you weren't in the study.

- There is always a chance that the experimental treatment can give you a worse result than the standard treatment.

How Can You Find Out About Ongoing Studies?

Most doctors treating prostate cancer do not participate in clinical studies nor are they aware of ones you might consider joining. You should not rely on your doctor to find a study for you. In some cases, they may not encourage you to join for financial reasons; they will lose out on the revenue they might have earned by taking care of you. The sad truth is most clinicians are not interested in research studies. Fortunately, many clinical trials are registered. You can find out about studies looking to recruit volunteers by visiting www.clinicaltrials.gov or www.cancer.gov/clinicaltrials. The second site allows you to search for a study according to the extent of your cancer and where you live. The Web sites usually provide information about who to contact to find out more about the study and whether you meet the requirements for enrolling.

The Bottom Line About Research Studies

Although joining a research study is not for everyone, the best thing you can do is get all the information about ongoing studies for your medical condition. If you find a study that interests you, do not hesitate to call one of the doctors conducting the study to learn about the details. They can discuss the advantages and disadvantages of signing up. Your family doctor may be a good resource to help you decide if you should enroll. Remember, many men who participate in a clinical study are helped and you might be, too.

New Hope on the Horizon

32

During the last few years, significant progress has occurred in the treatment of prostate cancer with the approval of several new drugs for men with metastatic disease. Other drugs and tests are showing encouraging results and may become available in the next few years. As you "surf" the Net, you are likely to read stories as new research gets reported. Some of them are still recruiting patients and you may be a good candidate. A description of the treatments undergoing testing in phase III studies and those awaiting a decision from the FDA is shown below in alphabetical order:

Abiraterone acetate is a pill that stops the production of testosterone. Preliminary studies show it may improve survival in men with metastatic disease even after having medical or surgical castration. It is being tested in men with advanced disease who have progressed while on hormone therapy. The study was recently stopped because the results showed the drug was beneficial and hopefully, this will lead to its approval by the FDA in the near future.

Alpharadin is a radioactive drug containing Radium-223 that is injected into the bloodstream and gets into bones invaded by prostate cancer. In phase II studies of men with metastatic prostate cancer who got worse while on hormone therapy, alpharadin showed an improvement in survival. It is now being tested in phase III studies.

313

Antivascular endothelial growth factor therapies. Most solid tumors like prostate cancer require a blood supply to grow. Cancer cells make proteins that tell the body to form new blood vessels. This process is called *angiogenesis*. One group of these proteins is called *vascular endothelial growth factors* (*VEGF*). Drugs that block these proteins may stop tumors from making new blood vessels. They are called *anti-VEGF therapies*. Limiting the blood supply may stop a cancer from growing. Several are currently Food and Drug Administration (FDA)-approved but none are for prostate cancer. Usually, they are too weak to be used alone. Studies are underway combining them with chemotherapy. The anti-VEGF drugs being tested for advanced prostate cancer include *bevacizumab* (*Avastin*), *sorafenib* (*Nexavar*), and *cediranib* (*AZD2171*).

Custirsen (OGX-011) blocks the production of a protein called *clusterin*, which is needed to keep cancer cells alive. In a phase II study, combining this drug with docetaxel showed a better survival than men getting docetaxel alone. It is being tested in combination with docetaxel and prednisone in men who have previously responded to docetaxel chemotherapy.

Denosumab is a drug recently approved to prevent bone fractures in women with osteoporosis. A Phase III study was done in men with bone metastases who were receiving hormone therapy to see if it would reduce *skeletal related events* or SRE's. That includes fractures, radiation or surgery to the bones and spinal cord compression. Denosumab did a significantly better job at preventing bone fractures than zoledronic acid. During one year of treatment, an SRE occurred in 41% of men on zoledronic acid compared to 36% on denosumab. The drug also delayed the time to the first SRE by almost 4 months compared to the zoledronic acid. The overall side effects were similar with the two treatments. The other advantages of Denosumab are that it is injected under the skin whereas zoledronic acid must be infused into a vein over 15 minutes and it does not require kidney function monitoring like zoledronic acid. The

FDA is expected to make its decision about denosumab for men with bone metastases very soon.

Estradiol patches deliver estrogen to the body with a reduced risk of causing heart attacks and the potential to avoid causing osteoporosis. Small studies suggest it might be another way to do medical castration. This treatment is being studied in England in men who need to begin hormone therapy for advanced prostate cancer and if the results are positive, studies may eventually be done in the United States.

High intensity focused ultrasound has been in use in several countries outside the United States for many years but it is not currently approved for use in the United States. Studies are in progress to determine its potential role in men with early stage disease by comparing it to men getting brachytherapy.

MDV3100 blocks male hormones from causing the growth of prostate cancer cells. It works differently than other hormone therapies currently in use. It is being tested in men with progressive metastatic disease who have previously been treated with hormone therapy and chemotherapy using docetaxel.

PCA3 urine test PCA3 is a gene that is present in about 90% of prostate cancers and can be measured in urine. It may be useful for deciding which men should have a repeat prostate biopsy after one is negative. The test is currently available in Europe and a decision is expected by the FDA for its use in the United States.

Toremifene (Acapodene) is an FDA-approved drug under the name Fareston for use in women with advanced breast cancer. It belongs to a group of drugs called *selective estrogen receptor modulators* (SERM) that can have an effect either similar to or opposite estrogen. Studies showed it has a positive effect in men on hormone therapy for prostate cancer by reducing fractures. It is under review by the FDA and a decision should be available soon.

Zibotentan (ZD4054) belongs to a group of drugs called *endothelin receptor antagonists* (ERA). *Endothelins* help cells grow and endothelin-receptor antagonists may stop that from occurring. Several phase III studies are underway in men with advanced disease. One of them recently failed to show it was effective when given to men with a rising PSA after medical or surgical castration for metastatic disease. Other studies are testing it in combination with docetaxel chemotherapy or by itself in men with less advanced disease.

Zoledronic acid (Zometa) is currently an approved drug for patients with prostate, breast, lung, and other solid tumors that have spread to the bones. It reduces the chance of developing a skeletal-related event such as a fracture. At present, this drug is more restricted in men with prostate cancer. The FDA-approval states that men must first show evidence that the cancer is getting worse despite hormone therapy before it is used. Testing is underway to find out if men benefit by getting the drug earlier in the disease.

Many drugs not described here are also being tested in phase I and phase II studies. Hopefully, the initial results will be positive leading to their continued development and eventual approval by the FDA.

VI

WHAT YOU CAN DO TO HELP YOURSELF

The Role of Complementary and Alternative Medicine

People who are ill often search for things they can do to help their condition, and prostate cancer is no exception. Surveys have found that more than one quarter of men with this disease do something on their own. That includes modifying their diet or taking some type of unconventional therapy such as herbs, vitamins, or dietary supplements. Other approaches used include yoga, exercise, massage, meditation, spiritual healing, and group counseling.

Eastern medicine has used herbs for thousands of years, with abundant testimonials from physicians, patients, and holistic care-givers praising their value. Laboratory or epidemiologic studies routinely are used to support their recommendations. Many people promote their use by saying, "Even if there is no good proof they work, perhaps they will help. Why not take them since they will not cause you any harm?"

The truth is, that may not be the case. Well-done studies have shown that some supplements are harmful. For example, good studies show that vitamin A increases the risk of dying from lung cancer in people who smoke and vitamin E can cause bleeding in the brain. Those results alone should make you think twice about claims that supplements are never harmful. Because the goal of this book is to tell you the strengths and weaknesses of all the things you can do for your cancer, the same will apply for these unconventional treatments. To help you decide what to do, each intervention discussed in this chapter will be assigned to one of the following groups based on the best available scientific information:

- Group I: Good studies show they definitely are helpful, meaning you *should strongly consider using them.*

- Group II: Uncontrolled studies show they might be helpful and do not cause harm. *Taking them is not unreasonable* if you are highly motivated to do something on your own.

- Group III: Laboratory or animal studies show there is some biological activity against cancer cells, but there is no way to tell what they would do to men with prostate cancer. Also, there is insufficient information to know if they might be harmful in some way or what dose should be used. This means *you probably should not use them* until better information becomes available about their safety.

- Group IV: Good studies show they do not help or they cause harm, which means *you definitely should not use them.*

The National Cancer Institute puts these interventions into the following five categories:

- Biologically based, which uses things occurring in nature such as diet, foods, herbs, and vitamins

- Whole medical systems such as Chinese medicine, homeopathy, or naturopathic medicine

- Mind-body medicine such as meditation, yoga, or hypnosis

- Body-based practices such as massage

- Energy medicine such as tai chi

What Should You Eat?

Diet definitely plays an essential role in our health. Our bodies need certain nutrients to function properly. Heart disease, diabetes, and obesity are clearly on the rise, in part because of poor nutrition. Diet is often used as one explanation for the much lower incidence of prostate cancer in Japan compared to the United States. Uncontrolled studies *suggest* that foods such as tomatoes, soy, red wine, and green tea reduce the chance of getting this disease. Other foods like fat and red meat *may* increase the risk of developing it or *may* make prostate cancer progress more quickly.

Many men are motivated to change their diet after they have been diagnosed with this disease. You already may have asked your doctor, "What should I eat?" or "Are any foods definitely good or bad for me?" Even though there is *no definite proof* that eating a certain way will help fight your cancer, there are other benefits. At a minimum, it can help you feel better, give you more strength and energy, and enable you to cope with some of the side effects caused by your treatment. The bottom line is good nutrition *may* improve your quality-of-life and help you in your battle against prostate cancer.

The importance of finding out if alternative therapies are beneficial has greatly increased because of the growing interest in active surveillance of prostate cancer. Currently, more than 60% of men diagnosed today have "low-risk" prostate cancer and most of them will not benefit from aggressive treatment. For many of them, active surveillance is hard to accept because they view it as "doing nothing." Active surveillance might become more acceptable if any of these "alternative" interventions can show a long-term benefit. Men would then feel that they are "doing something."

Medical journals contain many studies aimed at finding out if dietary and lifestyle changes are good for men with this disease. One well-done trial included 93 men with low-risk prostate cancer. They all chose to have active surveillance rather than immediate treatment. Men were then assigned to a control group that had no intervention or to a group that would get a "lifestyle program" consisting of the following:

- A vegan diet supplemented with soy, fish oil, vitamin E, selenium, and vitamin C

- Moderate exercise (walking 30 minutes six days a week)

- Stress management techniques (yoga, stretching, breathing, imagery relaxation for 60 minutes per day)

- A one-hour weekly support group meeting to encourage them to follow the program

The vegan diet was mostly fruits, vegetables, whole grains, legumes, and soy. Only 10% of calories were from fat. The results are shown in the next table.

Effect of Lifestyle Changes in Men With Prostate Cancer

Result	Control Group	Experimental Group
Average Prostate-specific antigen (PSA) level at start of study	6.4 ng/mL	6.2 ng/mL
Average PSA level after one year	6.7 ng/mL	6.0 ng/mL
Percentage of men getting surgery, radiation, or hormone therapy within one year	14%	0%
Average weight lost after one year	0 lb	10 lb

The study found that the group following the lifestyle changes had a slightly lower average PSA level after one year. Also, fewer men went off active surveillance. Usually, active surveillance is stopped when the PSA level rises or if other changes suggest that cancer is growing. That happened to six men in the control group but none in the experimental group.

Despite these early encouraging results, many questions still need to be answered. Will this intervention continue to prevent the disease from progressing? Will it help men avoid suffering from their cancer in the future? Is the entire program really needed or would some portion of it be enough to get the same benefit? For example, good studies have shown that vitamin E and selenium do not prevent prostate cancer. That might mean they also are not helping men who have the disease. Although it is far too early to draw any conclusions, the results are going in the right direction. If nothing else, men who make such changes seem to have a better quality-of-life and are not being harmed (group II).

Every five years, two government agencies publish *The Dietary Guidelines for Americans*, which contains general suggestions about diet for the general public. The last edition was in 2005 and the 2010 edition will be released very soon. It will be based on more scientific studies than in the past. All of them can be put into Group I. You can access this guideline and the new edition on the Internet for free at www.health.gov/dietaryguidelines/. Some of the recommendations from the 2005 and 2010 reports include the following:

- Overweight or obese adults should lose weight

- Consume 2,000 cal per day adjusted for your level of activity

- Eat two cups of fruit per day

- Eat 2½ cups of vegetables each day that includes dark green vegetables, orange, legumes, starch vegetables, and others

- Get less than 10% of calories from saturated fats, keep trans fats as low as possible, and eat less than 300 mg of cholesterol per day

- Keep total fat intake between 20% and 35% of total calories, mainly from fish, nuts, and vegetable oils

- Eat lean, low-fat, or fat-free meat and milk products

- Limit sodium intake to 1,500 mg per day

- Get essential nutrients from foods. Multivitamin and mineral supplements are discouraged

- Consume two servings of seafood per week to reduce the risk of dying from heart attacks

Until the new guideline is published, a good idea is for you to consult with a dietician who can review what you eat and make suggestions.

Although the Internet is full of "recommendations," the truth is that no diet has been shown to improve the outcome for men with prostate cancer. The reason some food items are being recommended by doctors is because extracts from these foods stopped or slowed the growth of prostate cancer cells growing in the laboratory. So far, however, no well-done studies have been done to know if any of these food products help men who have the disease. Uncontrolled studies in men show inconsistent results. Some of them showed the cancers were less aggressive in men with increased intake of these items and others showed no effect. The right amount needed is also unknown. A partial list of these foods includes fish oils, soy, tomatoes, broccoli, berries, pomegranate juice, cauliflower, watercress, cabbage, and other cruciferous vegetables. The good news is they are not harmful when taken in moderation and are part of a healthy diet (group II).

Soy contains several chemicals that show anticancer activity in laboratory studies. Some people believe soy intake is one reason Asian men have less prostate cancer than American men. Soy extracts sold in health food stores often are promoted for men with prostate cancer. Here too, uncontrolled studies show conflicting results. In one report, 20 men with recurrent prostate cancer drank soymilk three times a day for one year. Their PSA level increased more slowly than men that did not drink it. Without proper studies, no conclusions are possible. Foods containing soy do not appear to be harmful so incorporating them into your diet is quite reasonable. That may not be true for soy supplements (soy foods–group II, soy supplements–group III).

Garlic contains several ingredients including sulfur, arginine (an amino acid), isoflavones, and selenium. Consuming garlic has been recommended as a way to reduce the risk of some cancers, including prostate cancer. Although laboratory studies suggest that one of the ingredients in garlic blocks the growth of prostate cancer cells, no prospective studies have been done treating men with this disease. Several uncontrolled epidemiological studies looked at whether garlic intake prevented prostate cancer and the conclusions were mixed. Studies will be difficult to do in men with prostate cancer because of the varied ways garlic is prepared. It does have minor potential risks including heartburn, nausea, and it may be a blood thinner (foods–group II, supplements–group III).

Brazil nuts have been recommended because they contain high amounts of selenium. A government study in 2010 found that selenium did not prevent prostate cancer. No proper studies have been done in men with prostate cancer to know its effect. The only real downside to eating Brazil nuts is the high calorie content (group II).

Herbs and Other Dietary Supplements

Herbs are substances from plants that are used for medicines or for flavoring foods. Because many drugs in use today have come from this source, it seems logical that other untested herbs might also be helpful in treating this disease. Some of them have been shown to affect prostate cancer cells in laboratory experiments, but it is unknown whether they would have a similar effect in men with the disease. That has not stopped them from being promoted by alternative health books or anticancer Web sites. Because of the challenge of doing proper studies, companies sometimes "overstate" their case and promote a supplement inappropriately.

In 1994, Congress passed a law called the *Dietary Supplement Health and Education Act*. It sets certain rules about dietary supplements that include the following:

- They *must* be intended to supplement the diet.

- They *can* contain one or more herbs, vitamins, minerals, amino acids, or other botanical agents.

- They *are* to be taken by mouth as a tablet, powder, liquid, or capsule.

- They *must* be labeled as being a dietary supplement.

- They *do not require proof that they are safe or effective.*

- Companies may claim that a supplement supports health, can replace a deficiency, or can be related to a body function if research supports the claim.

- They *cannot make false claims about the effect.*

- They *must state, "It is not intended to diagnose, treat, cure, or prevent any disease."*

The last point is critical because many of the supplements on the market overstep this boundary. The Food and Drug Administration (FDA) is increasingly sending out warnings to companies about their claims. Keep this in mind when you consider taking a supplement based on claims made in magazines or on the Internet. The problem with many of these supplements is that little is known about their interaction with traditional medications. The government does not have the time or money to check out every claim. For that reason, *consult with your doctor before taking them. Be sure there is no added risk because of other medications you take.*

Two obstacles for finding out if herbs and supplements are useful is the high cost of doing proper studies and the difficulty in making money after the studies are done. Valid studies could take many years to complete because prostate cancer usually grows very slowly and companies would have difficulty getting an exclusive patent to sell the product.

To save time, some studies measure changes in the time it takes for the PSA to double in value as a way to tell if the cancer is being affected. Men with a long PSA doubling time are thought to be in less danger than those whose PSA doubles quickly. One European study assigned 42 men with a rising PSA level after radical prostatectomy or radiation to receive either a placebo or a supplement containing soy, isoflavones, lycopene, silymarin, and antioxidants. At the end of 10 weeks, the PSA doubling time in the group getting the supplements was 1,150 days compared to only 445 days in the control group. The study may be too small to make any conclusions. Although this is an encouraging result, the following questions need answering.

- What dose and preparation is needed of each supplement?

- Are all of them needed or could some of them be eliminated?

- What are the side effects?

- Do any of them interfere with other medications?

Longer follow-up is needed to determine if this supplement will improve survival or cause any side effects (group III).

The government Web site (www.nutrition.gov) is a useful resource for finding out about many alternative therapies. Information about other commonly used agents for prostate cancer or cancer in general, is included below.

Aloe vera has been used as a topical gel to reduce burns to the skin from radiation treatments. No good scientific studies have been done to support this claim (group III).

Astragalus has been used in Chinese medicine in combination with other herbs to boost the immune system. Almost all the available studies are from Chinese journals so their quality is difficult to evaluate. The herb is considered to be safe but little is known about its effect in prostate cancer patients. Studies are in progress to learn more about its effects (group II).

Bitter almond (Pygeum africanum) is often combined with saw palmetto to treat urinary problems in men. Laboratory studies show it inhibits the growth of prostate cancer cells. Although it appears safe in humans up to one year of use, there is no evidence that it has any effect in men with prostate cancer (group II).

Black cohosh has been used in women to treat hot flashes and other symptoms of menopause. It has also been suggested for men with hot flashes caused by hormone therapy. Supporting studies are lacking. Well-done studies have failed to show any improvement in hot flashes in women and some severe side effects have occurred, such as liver failure (group III).

Cat's claw has been used to help improve the immune system. It has not been well studied in men with prostate cancer. Little is known about its side effects or whether it interacts with other drugs (group III).

Echinacea has been recommended to treat and prevent colds. Because the immune system of cancer patients often is weakened, there is an increased risk for infections. Randomized studies testing three preparations showed no ability to prevent or shorten the duration of the common cold. No studies have been done in men with prostate cancer (group IV).

Ephedra has been use for weight loss, increased energy, and improved exercise performance. Although there is some evidence it can help men lose weight, the risk of stroke or heart attack is increased. In 2004, the FDA banned the sale of any supplement containing ephedra (group IV).

Evening primrose oil comes from the yellow flowers of a plant and contains an essential fatty acid. Normally, essential fatty acids must be obtained from our diet because our body can't make them. This supplement is made by putting the plant seeds into a capsule. It has been promoted for prostate health and to reduce inflammation, but no studies are available to assess whether it works or causes side effects (group III).

Flaxseed and flaxseed oil contains fiber, lignan, alpha-linolenic acid, and omega-3 fatty acids. It is used as a laxative and to lower cholesterol. Although it is frequently recommended for men with prostate cancer, no long-term studies have been done. A short-term study assigned men with localized prostate cancer to the following:

- a low-fat diet supplemented with 30 g per day of flaxseed

- a low-fat diet

- a regular diet supplemented with flaxseed

- a control group getting only a regular diet

All the men were followed for 21 days before having their prostate removed. The prostate glands were examined for the ability of the cancer cells to divide, which might be a crude measure of how well they grow. The study found that the cancer cells in the flaxseed-treated men did not divide as well as the controls or those taking only a low-fat diet. No side effects were reported. Because studies show that flaxseed can reduce absorption of drugs taken by mouth and limit their effectiveness, you should ask your doctor if it is safe for you. Although no conclusion can be made, these early results support doing more extensive studies (group II).

Genistein is one of the active ingredients in soy that is similar to human estrogen but much weaker. Estrogen is known to slow the growth of prostate cancer. In laboratory studies, genistein also slows the growth of prostate cancer cells. A prospective study was done in 16 men with prostate cancer on active surveillance. They were given genistein capsules three times per day for six months. At the end of the study, nine men had a stable or slightly lower PSA level. The genistein was stopped in 5% of the men because of diarrhea. The long-term benefits and side effects of genistein supplements are not yet known (group III).

Ginkgo biloba is commonly recommended to improve memory, mental function, and sexual function. Some Internet sites recommend ginkgo for patients with prostate cancer but they cite studies that do not really support that opinion. Well-done studies failed to show any improvement in memory. Side effects include an increased risk of bleeding and stomach problems. There are no prospective studies in men with prostate cancer (group III).

Ginseng is often promoted to boost the immune system. Laboratory studies found that two ingredients in this herb inhibited the growth of prostate cancer cells in the laboratory. According to the Web site of the National Institutes of Health (NIH), ginseng at recommended doses appears safe, although it may cause problems in diabetics. Its effect in men with prostate cancer is unknown (group II).

Goldenseal (yellow root) is an herb used by Native Americans for several health conditions. One of its ingredients is berberine, which stopped the growth of prostate cancer cells in a laboratory experiment. Although promoted on the Internet for the symptoms of prostate cancer, no clinical studies support this claim. The NIH states there is little information available about the safety of its long-term use at higher doses (group III).

Grape seed extract contains antioxidants. The NIH is funding studies to find out if it will prevent prostate cancer. One major ingredient is called *gallic acid*, which stopped prostate cancer cells from growing in the laboratory. It is well tolerated in humans, but no studies have been done to determine its effect in men with prostate cancer (group II).

Green tea is widely used in Asian countries and the United States and often is promoted for men with prostate cancer. It contains several chemicals called *catechins*. Laboratory experiments show that extracts of one of them called *epigallocatechin gallate* (EGCG) slowed the growth of prostate cancer in mice. In 2009, a review of published studies was unable to conclude that green tea prevents cancer. Also, no controlled studies have been done to know its effect in men with prostate cancer. Drinking a few cups of green tea per day appears safe, but some cases of liver toxicity have been reported with green tea extracts. Because it contains caffeine, it may cause difficulty sleeping and frequent urination. The safety of green tea extracts has not been well studied in men with prostate cancer (green tea–group II, green tea extracts–group III).

Licorice root extract contains ingredients that may slow the growth of cancer. A prospective, randomized study was started to determine the effect of combining licorice root with docetaxel in men with androgen-independent prostate cancer. Unfortunately, the study closed because not enough patients enrolled. This extract was one of the ingredients in PC-SPES (PC for prostate cancer and SPES meaning "hope" in Latin), an herbal mixture promoted years ago for patients with prostate cancer. PC-SPES is no longer available because the company making it was sued and went out of business when the product was found to contain estrogen. Licorice root extract combined with other herbs has also been tested in mice with prostate cancer and tumor growth was slowed. The safety of men taking it for more than a few weeks is unknown (group III).

Milk thistle has been used to reduce the growth of several tumors including prostate cancer. Two of its active ingredients, *silymarin* and *silybinin*, were found to inhibit the growth of prostate cancer cells and tumors in several laboratory studies. This may lead to testing in men with the disease. It does not appear to have major side effects (group II).

Mistletoe extract (Iscador) is widely used in Europe for cancer patients and many studies have been published although none included men with prostate cancer. The randomized studies found no benefit from the extract and many of the other studies were poorly done. The overall conclusion was that mistletoe extract *might* improve survival. Major side effects were not reported in the European studies and the NIH states that it is safe when used in proper doses. Its role in men with prostate cancer is unknown (group II).

Omega-3 fatty acids are widely recommended for their heart-health benefits. In 2006, a government agency reviewed all studies related to cancer and found no clear proof it prevented cancer. Uncontrolled studies suggested that men consuming low amounts of omega-3 fatty acids had a higher chance of getting aggressive prostate cancer and dying from the disease. However, no valid conclusions can be made. Because it has few side effects and appears to lower the risk of dying from heart disease, it may be worth taking. The evidence is strongest for fish and fish oil (fish and fish oil–group I, omega-3 supplements–group II).

Pomegranate juice contains many antioxidants. Some of its ingredients appear active against prostate cancer cells in laboratory experiments. That led to a prospective study in 46 men with a rising PSA level after being treated for prostate cancer. The PSA doubling time was determined before starting to drink 8 oz of pomegranate juice per day (made by POM Wonderful). A PSA test was repeated every three months. The juice was stopped if the PSA doubled or the cancer got worse. The PSA doubling time increased in 83% of the men during 56 months of treatment. Pomegranate juice did not reduce the testosterone level or cause any significant side effects. What conclusion can be made from this study? Unfortunately, it does not prove pomegranate juice helps men with prostate cancer. Presently, the FDA does not recognize changes in PSA as proof that a treatment is beneficial. In March and September 2010, the FDA warned POM Wonderful that its claim of slowing the progress of prostate cancer was a violation of the Federal Food Act. If you have a rising PSA level, taking 8 oz of pomegranate juice per day has some weak scientific support and does not appear to be harmful (group II).

Red clover belongs to a family of plants called *legumes*. Like soy, it contains *isoflavones*, which are active against prostate cancer cells in laboratory studies. One uncontrolled study gave red clover extract to 20 men in Australia a few weeks before they had a radical prostatectomy. An examination of their prostate gland showed more cancer cells had died compared to a group of men not receiving the extract. No studies have been done to see if red clover extract has any long-term benefit in men with this disease. It does appear safe when used for a short time (group II).

Saw palmetto (*Serenoa repens*) is a very popular herb promoted for treating symptoms of prostate enlargement. However, in 2006, a randomized study found it offered no improvement in men with moderate to severe urinary symptoms. In 2010, an extensive review of published studies also concluded that saw palmetto did not improve urinary symptoms. This herb also has no effect on PSA levels in men with urinary complaints. Although it does not cause serious side effects, it may affect the blood's ability to clot. At this time, there is no evidence that it benefits men with prostate cancer or those having urinary difficulties (group III).

Turmeric (circumin) is also called saffron and is commonly used to season Indian and Asian food. Laboratory studies found it slowed the growth of prostate cancers in mice. Although it is certainly safe to use, its effect in men with prostate cancer is unknown (group II).

Yohimbe is an herb from the bark of the yohimbe tree. It contains a chemical called *yohimbine*, which is sold as a prescription drug to treat men with erection problems. The amount of yohimbine in over-the-counter supplements is variable, its effectiveness is unknown, and significant side effects may occur (over the counter supplement-group III).

Zinc is an essential nutrient needed to make proteins and DNA. It is concentrated in the prostate gland and thought to help maintain a healthy prostate, but well-done studies have not been done. It can cause side effects at higher doses and can interact with some prescription drugs (group III).

Zyflamend is a mixture of ten herbs including holy basil, turmeric, ginger, green tea, rosemary, hu zhand, chinese goldthread, barberry, oregano and skullcap. Some studies *suggest* this mixture inhibits inflammation. It also shows activity against prostate cancer cells in laboratory experiments. A small study done in men with a high risk for prostate cancer showed it was not harmful but more studies are needed. In 2009, the FDA warned an Internet distributor about exaggerated claims. Zyflamend also has potential interactions with conventional drugs so you should discuss its safety with your doctor before taking it. (Group II).

Antioxidants

One reason given for how cancers develop is because of the effect of *free radicals*. They are unstable molecules that have the ability to alter normal cells, proteins, and DNA. *Antioxidants* are chemicals that stop free radicals from causing these changes, which protects the cells. Vitamin E and *selenium* are antioxidants that have been tested in randomized studies as preventive agents for prostate cancer. So far, they have not shown any benefit. Even though they do not prevent prostate cancer, could they possibly help men who already have the disease? The answer may be yes, but so far, not one well-done study has found any benefit. There is no evidence that they increase survival or help any other treatments be more effective. Until proper studies are done, the impact of these antioxidants will remain unknown.

Despite the lack of any studies showing they help, are they completely safe or could there by some harm from taking them? The following table shows the known side effects that may occur with these agents. Vitamin E in particular also may make chemotherapy less effective or increase the side effects of ketoconazole.

Side Effects of Antioxidant Vitamins

Antioxidant	Side Effects
Vitamin A	Fatigue, irritability, mental changes, anorexia, stomach discomfort, nausea, vomiting, mild fever, excessive sweating, thinning of the bones
Vitamin C	Nausea, vomiting, heartburn, stomach cramps, headache, an increased risk of bleeding, and kidney stones
Vitamin E	Fatigue, intestinal cramping, inflammation in veins, acne, diarrhea, increase in blood pressure in certain people, prolonged or increased risk of bleeding
Selenium	Nausea, vomiting, nail changes, loss of energy, irritability, loss of hair, inflammation of finger nails, fatigue, garlic breath odor, a metallic taste, muscle tenderness, shaking, lightheadedness, facial flushing, blood clotting problems, damage to liver and kidney, increase risk of diabetes

Another question about these vitamins is "What is the right dose?" Because no studies have compared different doses in men with prostate cancer, the answer remains unknown. Higher amounts certainly increase the risk of side effects. The bottom line is that so far, these vitamins have no proven benefit in men with prostate cancer and the information about their interaction with other drugs is limited (vitamins A and C, Selenium-group II, vitamin E-group III).

Lycopene is an antioxidant found in tomatoes, grapefruit, watermelon, and papaya that is active against prostate cancer in laboratory studies. It also is thought to reduce the risk of getting prostate cancer. A small prospective, randomized study was done in men scheduled to have a radical prostatectomy. For three weeks before surgery, 15 men were given lycopene and 11 men received no supplement. Although the study found fewer men in the lycopene group had cancer growing outside the prostate, the study groups were not balanced. This means the results do not prove lycopene was helpful. On the positive side, no side effects were reported. Further studies are needed to know if men with prostate cancer benefit from this supplement (group II).

Vitamin D deficiency occurs in many adults, particularly those who do not get enough outdoor exposure. This is thought to be a factor in the development of colon and breast cancer. Uncontrolled studies suggest a health benefit from maintaining a vitamin D level of 40 to 60 ng/mL. Blood tests are available to check your level. An intake of 2,000 IU per day of vitamin D3 is considered safe. No studies demonstrate a benefit from maintaining higher levels in men with prostate cancer, but it may be helpful for overall health (group II).

Homeopathy or Naturopathic Medicine

The idea behind homeopathy is to give small amounts of substances that in larger doses would cause the same symptoms as the disease being treated. This is supposed to result in patients "healing themselves." The FDA requires that homeopathic remedies can only be sold over the counter if they are promoted for minor health problems. If they are recommended to treat a more serious illness, like cancer, they must be sold by prescription. This whole field is controversial. Presently, there is no good evidence for a beneficial effect of homeopathy in men with prostate cancer and little is known about its side effects (grade III).

Mind–Body Medicine

The idea of this approach is to get the mind to help heal the body and lower stress. It includes meditation, yoga, hypnosis, and counseling. There is little evidence for any risks and they may reduce stress and improve quality-of-life. A study done in 10 men with a rising PSA level after radical prostatectomy looked at the effect of a stress-reduction program and a low-fat, plant-based diet on PSA levels over four months. The PSA doubling time increased in eight of them. It is unknown what role stress reduction played in this response or whether there is any long-term benefit. There is no evidence of any harm (group II).

The Bottom Line About Complementary Therapies

By now, you realize just how confusing this topic is. The fact is that little research has been done to know which, if any, interventions are truly good for men with prostate cancer. Until more is known, incorporating the items in group I and group II into your treatment plan is reasonable, providing you check first with your doctor. For now, the best and safest advice to give you is to avoid taking anything in groups III or IV. Remember, anyone who tells you these interventions are completely safe is not giving you the whole story. Still, you might decide to take some of them because the risks are acceptable to you. As with everything else in this book, the goal is to have you make an informed choice.

Using the Internet

34

One of the most profound changes for men with prostate cancer has been the explosion of information on the Internet. Typing in the words "prostate cancer" in a search engine in October 2010 gave more than 16 million "hits" or sites. No matter what aspect of the disease you want to know about, you will likely be over-whelmed with information. Right now, the Internet is a two-edged sword. It can provide you with very valuable and useful information, but it also can be inaccurate and biased. The challenge is to separate the good from the bad, which is not easily done.

Today, anyone can create a Web site relatively easily without having to meet any specific requirements. Documents on the World Wide Web are unregulated and unmonitored. As yet, no Internet police are available to check out each site for its accuracy. No rating service or "good housekeeping seal of approval" will identify the sites worth visiting. One day a site gives you the right information and then something changes making the information outdated and incorrect. Knowledge about prostate cancer is changing rapidly and few Internet sites are regularly updated. Even support group Web sites do not contain the most up-to-date information, so relying on them could give you the wrong information. Some Web sites appear balanced, unbiased, and accurate but the information they contain is three or four years old. In that case, you will need to make sure that nothing new has occurred to change the message.

338

One of the biggest concerns about using the Internet is that many of the Web sites are really marketing tools promoting doctors, hospitals, or company products. The way they present results seems appropriate, yet it is often biased and very misleading.

So where does this leave you? Should you avoid the Internet or embrace it? Are there things you can do or questions you can ask that will help you find the Web sites you can trust? The answer is yes. The place to begin is with sites that are organized and run by medical organizations or health agencies. Some examples include the following:

- The National Cancer Institute or NCI (http://www.cancer .gov/)—This site provides information about ongoing or completed research studies and general information about diagnosis and treatment of all cancers. It is generally up-to-date.

- The Center for Disease Control or CDC (http://cdc.gov/)— Provides a general overview of the treatment options for prostate cancer and other diseases.

- The Agency for Healthcare Research and Quality or AHRQ (http://ahqr.gov/)—Critically reviews medical topics with summaries based on good scientific methods.

Questions to Ask About an Internet Site

Your goal for every Web search is to find information that is accurate and up-to-date with little bias. Getting the answers to the following questions may help you decide if the information is trustworthy:

- Was the site created by a governmental or independent agency with no agenda other than to provide unbiased information?

- Is the author of the information identified with a description of his or her credentials, education, or experience, and is there a way to contact him or her?

- Was more than one person responsible for creating the information?

- Is the date the information was created clearly indicated so you can tell if it is current?

- Is the author, in any way, connected with or supported by a medical company that makes a product or treatment, which may suggest it is biased?

- Is the site promoting a doctor, hospital, clinic, or specific treatment that could indicate a bias?

- Are ads visible on the Web site promoting the treatment that is the focus of the topic being discussed?

In response to the need for unbiased up-to-date information, I have created a unique video Web site that can be accessed for free at www.prostatevideos.com. Each video is approximately five to seven minutes long. The Web site contains information about every aspect of the disease as if you and I were sitting across from each other having a conversation. Although it has not been put together with input from multiple doctors, it strictly follows the principles of good science. Like this book, it will tell you the pros and cons of all the options available for treating every stage of prostate cancer. A treatment will be recommended only if well-done studies clearly show it is better than the other options available. This Web site is meant to supplement what you read. Some people can understand certain things more easily when they hear it rather than read it. More than 100 videos on prostate cancer are available for your viewing. Old ones are updated and new ones are made when important new information becomes available. The site has received more than 175,000 visits in the past two years and you are encouraged to see if it contains additional information to help you with your treatment.

The Bottom Line About the Internet

If you are reading this book, then you are clearly interested in wanting to learn more about your disease than what your doctor has told you. The Internet can be a great aid but caution is needed so you will get the right information that can help you.

The Role of Support Groups and Counseling

35

The History of Prostate Cancer Support Groups

Most doctors treating men with prostate cancer have focused their time and effort on the "medical" aspects of the disease. They have searched for ways to improve survival and reduce the side effects of both the disease and the treatments. The good news is that many significant changes have occurred over the past 30 years. Although medical personnel have gotten better at treating prostate cancer, often they don't address the mental and emotional effects it has on men and their families.

You probably have heard about AA or Alcoholics Anonymous. It is a program for individuals trying to solve or control their problem with alcohol. It has helped countless individuals and continues to serve as an example of the benefits of a social interaction for people struggling with the same problem.

Over the last 20 years, support groups have evolved for people with various diseases including prostate cancer. Currently, one of the largest prostate cancer support groups in the United States is called Us TOO. It was started in 1990 in response to unmet needs by one of my own patients, Mr. Ed V. He had been treated with a new type of radiation therapy that caused him very severe problems with his bowels and his urinary control. Although every option was explored for treating those problems, he and his wife became anxious and depressed. They asked me, "Isn't anyone else having the same trouble? Aren't there other men and wives we can talk to about how they are dealing with these problems?"

After reading about the value of the breast cancer support group called Y-Me, it seemed to me that there clearly was an unmet need for men with prostate cancer. A short time later, I invited my patients with prostate cancer and their wives to a meeting I arranged at the University of Chicago. The executive director of the Y-Me woman's group was invited to talk about the purposes and benefits of patient support groups. Following that meeting, several of the attendees worked together to form the prostate cancer support group known as Us TOO.

It is now a tax-free corporation with a president/chief executive officer, an elected Board of Directors, awareness and fund-raising activities and support, education and advocacy programs. Their stated mission is to "Help men and their families make informed decisions about prostate cancer detection and treatment through support, education and advocacy." More than 325 Us TOO chapters have been set up with about 24 located in countries outside the United States. They have a free Web site (www.ustoo.org) that contains information about locating a local chapter and a monthly newsletter that contains information about the disease. Most chapters have a monthly meeting where they invite a guest speaker to talk on some aspect of the diagnosis or management of prostate cancer. After each meeting, attendees talk with each other and provide support.

Another large national support group is called Man to Man. It is coordinated through the American Cancer Society and has similar activities including a free Web site at www.acs.org.

What Support Groups Do

As the support groups have matured, their function has expanded. Some of the roles they play include the following:

- Providing men and their significant others with information about treatments that they were not told about or were not adequately explained by their doctor.

- Being a source of encouragement by seeing long-term survivors for those with a similar condition.

- Helping people express their feelings and cope with any emotional difficulties caused by the disease or side effects of the various treatments.

- Offering an opportunity to talk with men who have gone through the process of choosing a treatment and living with the results.

- Enabling women to share their experiences of coping with their partner's disease and its effect on their relationship.

Is There Anything Negative About Support Groups?

Ideally, a support group should result in nothing but benefits to those who attend. But participating in a support group does present some minor risks. The people who attend are often very passionate about what they believe is the "right" thing or "best" thing to do for various aspects of the disease. Someone who had a good result from his treatment may strongly encourage a newly diagnosed individual to choose that same treatment. They may fail to recognize why a different treatment might be more appropriate. Members of a support group are patients, not physicians, and they may be quite biased on how they present information. Sometimes they move beyond providing support and counseling to outright "recommending" treatment without accurately presenting the facts. They also tend to encourage the use of unconventional approaches such as herbs, vitamins, and supplements for treating the disease without an awareness of their limitations or risks.

The Bottom Line About Support Groups

Despite the potential limitations, support groups provide many important benefits. If you are aware of the possible biases, then attending one or more meetings will be worth your time.

Thousands of men and their significant others have benefitted from these groups. Although support groups may not be for everyone, you should know they exist, they are free to attend, they make newcomers feel comfortable, and they have no specific requirements that you "tell your story." Surprisingly, many doctors are still not tuned in to the benefits of attending a support group meeting. Many will not make you aware of them nor encourage you to attend. Generally, support groups can best be summed up by the motto: "Learning to cope through knowledge and hope."

Is There a Role for Counseling?

A diagnosis of prostate cancer is accompanied by many negative emotions including fear, anger, panic, and depression. Perhaps you already had trouble coping with changes in your sexual function before your cancer was detected. Prostate cancer treatment brings another set of emotions depending on what was done to you and whether any side effects occurred. Confronting those feelings is something you may have not faced before and it can affect your quality-of-life.

If you are having any emotional or psychological difficulties, what should you do? The first and best advice is *don't despair*. Psychiatrists, psychologists, and social workers are trained to help you cope. The best advice you can get is to be open to the idea of seeking out one of them. There is nothing wrong with your deciding to get help for these emotions. Short-term depression and anxiety are common among men with prostate cancer, yet few doctors will ask about it or suggest seeing a therapist. Antidepressants and other medications can be very helpful especially while you try to decide which treatment is right for you. Many men begin to feel better after they have been treated. Their need for medication or counseling decreases or goes away. Your partner also may be struggling, worrying about your life being cut short. She, too, can also benefit from counseling. The best advice is to confront your feelings rather than avoid them, and keep an open dialogue with your partner so you can help each other get through it. Then you can resume living again. If you have specific concerns about your disease, make sure to discuss them with your doctor. Not uncommonly, men think they are in greater danger than is really the case. That certainly increases the level of anxiety. The bottom line is to realize that a diagnosis of prostate cancer can cause a lot of distress but psychological support is available and beneficial.

What to Do When Therapy Is No Longer Effective

Despite all the available treatments, some men eventually will die from their prostate cancer. A difficult decision is when to stop receiving medications that are not successfully fighting the cancer and accept what is going to happen sooner rather than later. No one can tell you when that should be done because it is a very personal decision. But when it happens, the goals change from trying to live as long as possible to controlling pain, maintaining quality-of-life, and learning to accept what is happening.

The Role of Hospice

Hospice is not so much a place to go for medical care as it is a concept. The word hospice means "guesthouse" in Latin, but in the 1960s a British doctor started a team approach to delivering care that included modern pain control methods for people nearing death. In 1974, the first hospice began in the United States, and today it provides invaluable services to people who are at the end stages of their lives. Hospice is composed of a team of professionals including physicians, nurses, aides, social workers, counselors, therapists, spiritual caregivers, and volunteers. Although patients can be cared for at an inpatient location, hospice mostly provides services at home. Two of its advantages are the ability to remain in the comfort of your own home and have family members and friends present at all times. This is far better than the impersonal environment of a hospital.

When a patient enters hospice, they stop all the treatments aimed at trying to prolong their life and instead focus on feeling as good as possible for as long as possible. Without hospice, pain is often not adequately controlled. The drugs prescribed by many physicians may keep you comfortable for a few hours but not for all 24 hours of the day. The goal of hospice is to provide comfort and support while making sure that pain is completely eliminated or at least greatly reduced. Hospice workers will train someone from your home to make sure you get your medication. There is no reason anyone should endure even one hour of pain when medications are available that can eliminate or reduce it.

Controlling pain is not simply a matter of prescribing a pill. The best results come from titrating the pain medication, which means gradually increasing the dose or combining different drugs until the right amount is found. Narcotics often play a necessary role and you should not worry about taking them out of fear of becoming addicted. If those are the only drugs that eliminate the pain, then using them is the right thing to do.

Many men develop breakthrough pain, which means the drugs control the pain for a few hours but it returns before the next dose is due. A second drug is often very helpful in those cases. Adding an NSAID, a nonsteroidal anti-inflammatory drug, can prevent pain from recurring before another narcotic is taken. It can also reduce the need to raise the dose of the narcotic being used. The following are examples of some of the more common over-the-counter NSAIDs:

- ibuprofen

- Motrin

- Naprosyn

- Aleve

- aspirin

One mistake patients often make is waiting to take their medication until *after* their pain returns. A better approach is to take a drug *before* the pain develops because it helps keep a person pain free for a greater part of the day and night. The bottom line is no one should have to endure pain without making every effort to control it, and hospice staff is very experienced at doing that.

Pain is not the only symptom you may face. Depression, constipation, diarrhea, urinary leakage, and shortness of breath can happen and hospice staff will help address those as well.

When Should You Consult With Hospice?

A good time to consult with hospice is before it is needed. You can be receiving chemotherapy or other treatments and still be evaluated by a member of the hospice staff. The value of that approach is it will make for a smoother, more rapid transition when you decide the time is right. On average, men with prostate cancer spend the last six months of their lives in hospice.

What to Do When the End Is Near

In 1969, Elisabeth Kübler-Ross wrote a book called "On Death and Dying." She suggested that there were five stages of coping with grief that dying patients usually progressed through near the end of their lives. They are as follows:

- Denial. People feel like "This can't be happening, not to me."

- Anger. "This is not fair, why is it happening to me?"

- Bargaining. "Just let me live a little longer so I can see my grandchildren graduate from school."

- Depression. "I'm so sad, why go on? I know I am dying so why delay it?"

- Acceptance. "It's going to be okay. I can't fight it, I may as well prepare for it."

These stages do not always happen in this order and not everyone goes through every stage but the last one is very important. When a man with prostate cancer denies what is happening, it often will create a separation between him and his family. A healthier approach is to get to a point where one's feelings can be discussed with friends and family. Filling your remaining months, weeks, and days communicating with family and friends, doing those things that bring some pleasure, and reminiscing about pleasurable moments of your life can be a way to achieve an inner peace when the end finally arrives.

Glossary

adjuvant therapy—General term for giving a second treatment after another treatment has been completed.

alpha-blockers—Drugs that relax muscle cells in the prostate resulting in improvement in the urine stream and less nighttime urination.

5-alpha reductase inhibitors (5-ARIs)—Group of drugs that prevent normal prostate cells from converting testosterone to dihydrotestosterone.

alprostadil—Drug injected into the side of the penis or placed inside the tip of the penis as a suppository that creates an erection.

androgen ablation—General term for lowering or blocking the male hormone, testosterone.

androgen deprivation therapy (ADT)—A therapy in which male hormones in the body are taken away.

androgen-independent prostate cancer (AIPC)—Prostate cancer cells that do not depend on androgen for growth.

androstenediol—Chemical produced in the adrenal glands that can be converted by the body into testosterone.

androstenedione—Chemical produced in the adrenal gland that can be converted to testosterone.

androsterone—Male hormone made in the liver from the metabolism of testosterone.

antiandrogen—Drug that blocks hormone receptors that aid prostate cancer growth.

antiandrogen withdrawal (AAWD) phenomenon—Unusual response in which tumor cell growth slows rather than increases when antiandrogen drugs are stopped.

anticholinergic—Drugs that are used to treat overactive bladder.

antigen—Substance that causes the immune system to produce antibodies.

angiogenesis—Process of forming new blood vessels.

benign prostate hypertrophy (BPH)—Enlargement of the prostate gland.

bilateral adrenalectomy—Surgical removal of both adrenal glands.

bilateral orchiectomy (also bilateral orchidectomy)—Surgical removal of both testicles.

bound prostate-specific antigen (PSA)—Form of PSA that binds to proteins circulating in the bloodstream.

bowel fistula—Opening in the rectum that allows bowel contents to leak out.

capsular penetration—Cancer cells growing outside the capsule of the prostate.

combined androgen blockade (CAB)—Type of prostate cancer hormone therapy that combines lowering the testosterone and blocking male hormones from the adrenal gland.

corpus cavernosum—Pair of cylinder-shaped rods in the penis containing many blood vessels that fill with blood during an erection.

corpus spongiosum—Spongy tissue surrounding the male urethra within the penis that fills with blood during sexual stimulation.

cryoablation (also cryotherapy)— Process that uses extreme cold to destroy cells.

dihydrotestosterone (DHT)—Potent male hormone formed from testosterone by the enzyme 5-alpha reductase.

DNA—Abbreviation for deoxyribonucleic acid that contains all the genetic material found in every living cell.

dry orgasm—The tubes carrying seminal fluid to the penis have been cut preventing any fluid from coming out during an orgasm.

dysuria—Pain during urination.

endothelin receptor antagonists—Drug that blocks endothelin receptors.

endothelins—Proteins that constrict blood vessels.

erythropoietin—Hormone produced by the kidney that promotes the formation of red blood cells in the bone marrow.

erythropoietin-stimulating agents (ESAs)—Synthetic drugs that stimulate the body to form new red blood cells.

extracapsular extension—Prostate cancer cells growing outside the prostate capsule into the surrounding tissues.

follicle-stimulating hormone (FSH)—Hormone produced in the brain that helps sperm cells grow and mature.

free prostate-specific antigen (PSA)—Chemical forms of PSA that circulate in the bloodstream without binding to other proteins.

frozen section—Method used to process surgical specimens immediately by freezing the tissue.

genistein—Chemical that inhibits the formation of new blood vessels in the body.

gonadotropin-releasing hormone (GnRH) antagonist—Drug that stops the body from releasing hormones from the brain that normally play a role in sexual function, sperm production and stimulating prostate cancer cells without producing a temporary rise in testosterone.

gray (GY)—Metric term used to measure radiation units.

gynecomastia—Enlargement of the breasts.

half-life—Number of days required for 50% of the radiation to disappear from radioactive material.

high-grade prostatic intraepithelial neoplasia (HGPIN)—Abnormal prostate cells that have some features of cancer cells.

hormone deprivation—The process of taking away male hormones in the body.

hormone refractory prostate cancer—Prostate cancer that has progressed despite a reduction in the testosterone level in the body.

intensity-modulated radiation therapy (IMRT)—Method for delivering radiation that divides one large beam into many narrow beams.

intermittent androgen deprivation (IAD)—Treatment that involves repeatedly reducing the testosterone level and then allowing it to rise again.

intramuscular (IM)—Delivering medication by injecting it into a large muscle.

Kegel exercises—Method for strengthening the pelvic muscles that form part of the pelvic floor.

leukopenia—Drop in the number of white blood cells.

leukopheresis—Process of collecting blood, separating out certain types of cells, and then immediately returning the red blood cells back into the patient.

lithotomy position—Surgical position in which patients are laid on their back with knees bent, positioned above the hips, and spread apart using stirrups.

luteinizing hormone (LH)—Hormone produced in the pituitary gland of the brain that stimulates testosterone production in the testicles.

luteinizing hormone-releasing hormone (LHRH)—Hormone produced in a region of the brain called the hypothalamus, which plays a role in controlling testosterone in the body.

luteinizing hormone-releasing hormone agonist—Drugs that prevent the release of luteinizing hormone from the brain leading to a short-term increase in testosterone followed by a reduction in the production of testosterone.

luteinizing hormone-releasing hormone antagonist—Drugs that also prevent the release of luteinizing hormone from the brain leading to a reduction in the production of testosterone without causing a rise in testosterone.

luteinizing hormone-releasing hormone (LHRH) receptors— Area in the pituitary where luteinizing hormone-releasing hormone binds leading to the release of luteinizing hormone.

lycopene—Antioxidant found in tomatoes, grapefruit, watermelon, and papaya.

lymphocele—Collection of fluid following the removal of lymph nodes from the body.

maximum androgen blockade (MAB)—Type of prostate cancer hormone therapy that combines lowering the testosterone and blocking male hormones from the adrenal gland.

metabolic syndrome—Several changes occurring in response to a lowered testosterone that contributes to heart disease such as increases in cholesterol, low-density lipoproteins, and triglycerides.

nadir—In men with prostate cancer, usually refers to the lowest PSA level or testosterone level attained in response to treatment.

neutropenia—Decrease in the number of neutrophils, a specific type of white blood cell.

Partin tables—Series of tables that uses PSA, Gleason score, and clinical stage to predict the odds of having prostate cancer in the lymph nodes, seminal vesicles, or tissues outside the prostate.

penile implant—Artificial devices placed inside the penis that creates erections.

perineum—Area located around the rectal area of the body.

peripheral edema—Fluid accumulating in the tissues leading to swelling in the lower part of the body.

peripheral neuropathy—Feeling of burning or tingling in the fingers and toes.

ploidy analysis—Test that measures the amount of DNA contained in cells.

priapism—Erection that persists for several hours without sexual stimulation and requires medical intervention for it to be resolved.

prostate bed—Tissue in front of the rectum where the prostate gland originally was located prior to surgical removal.

prostatic acid phosphatase—Enzyme produced by the prostate, sometimes used to determine the extent of prostate cancer.

protein-specific antigen (PSA) bounce—Unexpected increase in the PSA level following radiation that is not caused by prostate cancer.

protein-specific antigen velocity (PSAV)—Speed at which the PSA level is rising in the bloodstream.

proton—Subatomic particle with an electric charge found in the nucleus of an atom.

radiation absorbed dose (rad)—Metric term used for measuring the amount of radiation absorbed by the body.

retrograde ejaculation—The absence of fluid coming out from the tip of the penis after an orgasm during sexual stimulation.

secondary Gleason grade—A number given to the second most common type of prostate cancer cells seen on a prostate biopsy.

subcutaneously (SubQ)—Method for delivering drugs by injecting them under the skin.

testosterone escape—Increase in the testosterone level above the castrate range of 50 ng/dL.

thrombocytopenia—Drop in the number of platelets in the bloodstream.

TNM system—Method to define the location of tumor in the body that assigns a T stage for the amount in the prostate gland, an N stage for the amount in the lymph nodes, and an M stage for the extent in other parts of the body.

total androgen blockade—Therapy used to eliminate or block the male sex hormones in the body coming from the testicles and adrenal glands.

transperineal biopsy—Prostate biopsy that is performed by passing needles through the skin in the perineal area and directing them into the prostate.

transrectal biopsy—Prostate biopsy performed by passing needles through the rectal wall and directing them into the prostate.

transurethral resection prostatectomy (TURP)—Operation performed through the urethra to remove the inner portion of the prostate.

tumor grade—Method for defining the appearance of cancer cells when viewed under the microscope.

tumor stage—Method for describing the location of cancer cells in the body.

ultrasensitive prostate-specific androgen (PSA)—Test to detect every amount of PSA in a blood sample.

urethral sloughing—Prostate tissue dies and falls into the urethra, sometimes leading to an inability to urinate.

urethral stricture—Scar that forms in the tube carrying urine from the bladder out through the tip of the penis.

valsalva maneuver—Increase in intraabdominal pressure created by straining.

vascular endothelial growth factors (VEGFs)—Chemical that stimulates the growth of new blood vessels.

Bibliography

Chapter 1

1. Lippman SM, Klein EA, Goodman PJ, et al. Effect of selenium and vitamin E on risk of prostate cancer and other cancers: the selenium and vitamin E cancer prevention trial (SELECT). JAMA. 2009;301(1):39–51.

2. Thompson IM, Goodman PJ, Tangen CM, et al. The influence of finasteride on the development of prostate cancer. N Engl J Med. 2003;349(3):215–224.

3. Kramer BS, Hagerty KL, Justman S, et al. Use of 5-alpha-reductase inhibitors for prostate cancer chemoprevention: American Society of Clinical Oncology/American Urological Association 2008 clinical practice guideline. J Clin Oncol. 2009;27(9):1502–1516.

4. Andriole GL, Bostwick DG, Brawley OW et al. Effect of dutasteride on the risk of prostate cancer. N Engl J Med. 2010;362:1192–1202.

Chapter 2

1. Andriole GL, Crawford ED, Grubb RL III, et al. Mortality results from a randomized prostate-cancer screening trial. N Engl J Med. 2009;360(13): 1310–1319.

2. Hugosson J, Carlsson S, Aus G, et al. Mortality results from the Göteborg randomised population-based prostate-cancer screening trial. Lancet Oncol. 2010;11(8):725–732.

3. Schröder FH, Hugosson J, Roobol MJ, et al. Screening and prostate cancer mortality in a randomized European study. N Engl J Med. 2009; 360(13):1320–1328.

Chapter 3

1. Catalona WJ, Smith DS, Wolfert RL, et al. Evaluation of percentage of free serum prostate-specific antigen to improve specificity of prostate cancer screening. JAMA. 1995;274(15):1214–1220.

2. Steward CS, Leibovich BC, Weaver AL, et al. Prostate cancer diagnosis using a saturation needle biopsy technique after previous negative sextant biopsies. J Urol. 2001;166(1):86–92.

3. Aboseif S, Shinohara K, Weidner N, et al. The significance of prostatic intra-epithelial neoplasia on prostate needle biopsy. Br J Urol. 1995;76:355–359.

Chapter 5

1. Michalski JM, Roach M III, Merrick G, et al. ACR appropriateness criteria on external beam radiation therapy treatment planning for clinically localized prostate cancer expert panel on radiation oncology—prostate. Int J Radiat Oncol Biol Phys. 2009;74(3):667–672.

2. National Cancer Institute Web site, 2010. Available at: http://www.cancer.gov. Accessed October 2010.

Chapter 6

1. Epstein JI, Allsbrook WC Jr, Amin MB, Egevad LL. Update on the Gleason grading system for prostate cancer: results of an international consensus conference of urologic pathologists. Adv Anat Pathol. 2006;13(1):57–59.

2. Ohori M, Wheeler TM, Scardino PT. The new American joint committee on cancer and international union against cancer TNM classification of prostate cancer. Cancer. 1994;74(1):104–114.

Chapter 7

1. Owens D, Lohr K, Atkins D, et al. AHRQ series paper 5: Grading the strength of a body of evidence when comparing medical interventions: AHRQ and the effective health-care program. J Clin Epidemiol. 2010;63(5):513–523.

Chapter 9

1. Lu-Yao GL, Albertsen PC, Moore DF, et al. Outcomes of localized prostate cancer following conservative management. JAMA. 2009;302(11): 1202–1209.

2. Bill-Axelson A, Holmberg L, Ruutu M, et al. Radical prostatectomy versus watchful waiting in early prostate cancer. N Engl J Med. 2005;352(19): 1977–1984.

3. Albertsen PC, Hanley JA, Fine J. 20-year outcomes following conservative management of clinically localized prostate cancer. *JAMA.* 2005; 293(17):2095–2101.

4. Bill-Axelson A, Holmberg L, Filén FJ, et al. Radical prostatectomy versus watchful waiting in localized prostate cancer: the Scandinavian prostate cancer group-4 randomized trial. *J Natl Cancer Inst.* 2008;100(16):1144–1154.

Chapter 10

1. Bastian PJ, Carter BH, Bjartell A, et al. Insignificant prostate cancer and active surveillance: from definition to clinical implications. *Eur Urol.* 2009;55:1321–1330.

2. Shappley WV III, Kenfield SA, Kasperzyk JL, et al. Prospective study of determinants and outcomes of deferred treatment or watchful waiting among men with prostate cancer in a nationwide cohort. *J Clin Oncol.* 2009;27(30):4980–4985.

3. Klotz L, Zhang L, Lam A, Nam R, Mamedov A, Loblaw A. Clinical results of long-term follow-up of a large, active surveillance cohort with localized prostate cancer. *J Clin Oncol.* 2010;28(1):126–131.

Chapter 11

1. Potosky AL, Davis WW, Hoffman RM, et al. Five-year outcomes after prostatectomy or radiotherapy for prostate cancer: the prostate cancer outcomes study. *J Natl Cancer Inst.* 2004;96(18):1358–1367.

2. Hoffman RM, Hunt WC, Gilliland FD, Stephenson RA, Potosky AL. Patient satisfaction with treatment decisions for clinically localized prostate carcinoma. Results from the Prostate Cancer Outcomes Study. *Cancer.* 2003;97(7):1653–1662.

3. Han M, Partin AW, Zahurak M, Piantadosi S, Epstein JI, Walsh PC. Biochemical (prostate-specific antigen) recurrence probability following radical prostatectomy for clinically localized prostate cancer. *J Urol.* 2003;169(2):517–523.

4. Wilt TJ, Macdonald R, Rutks I, Shamliyan TA, Taylor BC, Kane RL. Systematic review: comparative effectiveness and harms of treatments for clinically localized prostate cancer. *Ann Intern Med.* 2008;148(6): 435–448.

5. Hu JC, Gu X, Lipsitz SR, et al. Comparative effectiveness of minimally invasive vs open radical prostatectomy. *JAMA.* 2009;302(14):1557–1564.

6. Alibhai SM, Leach M, Tomlinson G, et al. 30-day mortality and major complications after radical prostatectomy: influence of age and comorbidity. *J Natl Cancer Inst.* 2005;97(20):1525–1532.

7. Thompson IM, Tangen CM, Paradelo J, et al. Adjuvant radiotherapy for pathological T3N0M0 prostate cancer significantly reduces risk of metastases and improves survival: long-term followup of a randomized clinical trial. *J Urol.* 2009;181(3):956–962.

Chapter 12

1. Heidenreich A, Ohlmann CH, Polyakov S. Anatomical extent of pelvic lymphadenectomy in patients undergoing radical prostatectomy. *Eur Urol.* 2007;52(1):29–37.

2. Messing EM, Manola J, Yao J, et al. Immediate versus deferred androgen deprivation treatment in patients with node-positive prostate cancer after radical prostatectomy and pelvic lymphadenectomy. *Lancet Oncol.* 2006;7(6):472–479.

Chapter 13

1. Kumar S, Shelley M, Harrison C, Coles B, Wilt TJ, Mason MD. Neoadjuvant and adjuvant hormone therapy for localised and locally advanced prostate cancer. *Cochrane Database Syst Rev.* 2006;(4):CD006019.

2. Pilepich MV, Caplan R, Byhardt RW, et al. Phase III trial of androgen suppression using goserelin in unfavorable-prognosis carcinoma of the prostate treated with definitive radiotherapy: report of Radiation Therapy Oncology Group Protocol 85-31. *J Clin Oncol.* 1997;15(3): 1013–1021.

3. Viani GA, Stefano EJ, Afonso SL. Higher-than-conventional radiation doses in localized prostate cancer treatment: a meta-analysis of randomized, controlled trials. *Int J Radiat Oncol Biol Phys.* 2009;74(5):1405–1418.

4. Agency for Healthcare Research and Quality. Comparative evaluation of radiation treatments for clinically localized prostate cancer: an update. Aug 2010. Available at http://www.cms.gov/coveragegeninfo/downloads/id69ta.pdf.

Chapter 14

1. Agency for Healthcare Research and Quality. Comparative effectiveness of therapies for clinically localized prostate cancer. Available at: http://effectivehealthcare.ahrq.gov/healthInfo.cfm?infotype=rr&ProcessID=9&DocID=79. Accessed October 2010.

2. Frank SJ, Grimm PD, Sylvester JE, et al. Interstitial implant alone or in combination with external beam radiation therapy for intermediate-risk prostate cancer: a survey of practice patterns in the United States. *Brachytherapy*. 2007;6(1):2–8.

3. Herstein A, Wallner K, Merrick G, et al. I-125 versus Pd-103 for low-risk prostate cancer: long-term morbidity outcomes from a prospective randomized multicenter controlled trial. *Cancer*. 2005;11(5):385–389.

4. Zelefsky MJ, Zaider M. Low-dose-rate brachytherapy for prostate cancer: preplanning vs intraoperative planning—intraoperative planning is best. *Brachytherapy*. 2006;5(3):143–144.

5. Ragde H, Korb LJ, Elgamal AA, Grado GL, Nadir BS. Modern prostate brachytherapy. Prostate specific antigen results in 219 patients with up to 12 years of observed follow-up. *Cancer*. 2000;89(1):135–141.

6. Miller DC, Sanda MG, Dunn RL, et al. Long-term outcomes among localized prostate cancer survivors: health-related quality-of-life changes after radical prostatectomy, external radiation, and brachytherapy. *J Clin Oncol*. 2005;23(12):2772–2780.

7. Filocamo MT, Li Marzi V, Del Popolo G, et al. Effectiveness of early pelvic floor rehabilitation treatment for post-prostatectomy incontinence. *Eur Urol*. 2005;48(5):734–738.

Chapter 15

1. Thompson I, Thrasher JB, Aus G, et al. Guideline for the management of clinically localized prostate cancer: 2007 update. *J Urol*. 2007;177(6):2106–2131.

2. Babaian RJ, Donnelly B, Bahn D, et al. Best practice statement on cryosurgery for the treatment of localized prostate cancer. *J Urol*. 2008;180(5):1993–2004.

3. Ellis DS, Manny TB Jr, Rewcastle JC. Cryoablation as a primary treatment for localized prostate cancer followed by penile rehabilitation. *Urology*. 2007;69(2):306–310.

4. Prepelica KL, Okeke Z, Murphy A, Katz AE. Cryosurgical ablation of the prostate: high risk patient outcomes. *Cancer.* 2005;103(8):1625–1630.

5. Hubosky SG, Fabrizio MD, Schellhammer PF, Barone BB, Tepera CM, Given RW. Single-center experience with third-generation cryosurgery for management of organ-confined prostate cancer: critical evaluation of short-term outcomes, complications, and patient quality-of-life. J *Endourol.* 2007;21(12):1521–1531.

6. Bahn DK, Lee F, Badalament R, Kumar A, Greski J, Chernick M. Targeted cryoablation of the prostate: Seven year outcomes in the primary treatment of prostate cancer. *Urology.* 2002;60(2 suppl 1):3–11.

Chapter 16

1. Levine GN, D'Amico AV, Berger P, et al. Androgen-deprivation therapy in prostate cancer and cardiovascular risk: a science advisory from the American Heart Association, American Cancer Society, and American Urological Association. *CA Cancer J Clin.* 2010;60(3): 194–201.

2. Studer UE, Collette L, Whelan P, et al. Using PSA to guide timing of androgen deprivation in patients with T0-4 N0-2 M0 prostate cancer not suitable for local curative treatment (EORTC 30891). *Eur Urol.* 2008;53(5):941–949.

3. Braga-Basaria M, Dobs AS, Muller DC, et al. Metabolic syndrome in men with prostate cancer undergoing long-term androgen-deprivation therapy. J *Clin Oncol.* 2006;24(24):3979–3983.

4. Salminen EK, Portin RI, Koskinen A, Helenius H, Nurmi M. Associations between serum testosterone fall and cognitive function in prostate cancer patients. *Clin Cancer Res.* 2004;10(22):7575–7582.

5. The Medical Research Council Prostate Cancer Working Party Investigators Group. Immediate versus deferred treatment for advanced prostatic cancer: initial results of the medical research council trial. *Br J Urol.* 1997;79(2):235–246.

6. Studer UE, Whelan P, Albrecht W, et al. Immediate or deferred androgen deprivation for patients with prostate cancer not suitable for local treatment with curative intent: European Organisation for Research and Treatment of Cancer (EORTC) Trial 30891. J *Clin Oncol.* 2006;24(12):1868–1876.

Chapter 17

1. Colombel M, Poissonnier L, Martin X, Gelet A. Clinical results of the prostate HIFU project. *Eur Urol Supplements*. 2006;5(6):491–494.

2. Poissonnier L, Chapelon JY, Rouvière O, et al. Control of prostate cancer by transrectal HIFU in 227 patients. *Eur Urol*. 2007;51(2):381–387.

Chapter 18

1. Chen RC, Clark JA, Manola J, Talcott JA. Treatment 'mismatch' in early prostate cancer: do treatment choices take patient quality-of-life into account? *Cancer*. 2008;112(1):61–68.

2. Penson DF, Feng Z, Kuniyuki A, et al. General quality-of-life 2 years following treatment for prostate cancer: what influences outcomes? Results from the prostate cancer outcomes study. *J Clin Oncol*. 2003;21(6):1147–1154.

3. Gore JL, Kwan L, Lee SP, Reiter RE, Litwin MS. Survivorship beyond convalescence: 48-month quality-of-life outcomes after treatment for localized prostate cancer. *J Natl Cancer Inst*. 2009;101(12):888–892.

4. Miller DC, Sanda MG, Dunn RL, et al. Long-term outcomes among localized prostate cancer survivors: health-related quality-of-life changes after radical prostatectomy, external radiation, and brachytherapy. *J Clin Oncol*. 2005;23(12):2772–2780.

5. Steineck G, Helgesen F, Adolfsson J, et al. Quality-of-life after radical prostatectomy or watchful waiting. *N Engl J Med*. 2002;347(11):790–796.

Chapter 19

1. Goldstein I, Lue TF, Padma-Nathan H, et al. Oral sildenafil in the treatment of erectile dysfunction. 1998. *J Urol*. 2002;167(2 pt 2):1197–1203.

2. Masson P, Lampert SM, Brown M, Shabsigh R. PDE-5 inhibitors: current status and future trends. *Urol Clin North Am*. 2005;32(4):511–525.

3. Mulhall JP, Ahmed A, Branch J, Parker M. Serial assessment of efficacy and satisfaction profiles following penile prosthesis surgery. *J Urol*. 2003;169(4):1429–1433.

4. Haab F, Trockman BA, Zimmern PE, Leach GE. Quality-of-life and continence assessment of the artificial urinary sphincter in men with minimum 3.5 years of followup. *J Urol*. 1997;158(2):435–439.

Chapter 20

1. Caloglu M, Ciezki J. Prostate-specific antigen bounce after prostate brachytherapy: review of a confusing phenomenon. *Urology.* 2009;74(6):1183–1190.

2. Freedland SJ, Humphreys EB, Mangold LA, et al. Risk of prostate cancer–specific mortality following biochemical recurrence after radical prostatectomy. *JAMA.* 2005;294(4):433–439.

3. Roach M III, Hanks G, Thames H Jr, et al. Defining biochemical failure following radiotherapy with or without hormonal therapy in men with clinically localized prostate cancer: recommendations of the RTOG-ASTRO Phoenix Consensus Conference. *Int J Radiat Oncol Biol Phys.* 2006; 65(4):965–974.

4. Jhaveri FM, Zippe CD, Klein EA, Kupelian PA. Biochemical failure does not predict overall survival after radical prostatectomy for localized prostate cancer: 10-year results. *Urology.* 1999;54(5):884–890.

Chapter 21

1. Freedland SJ, Partin AW, Humphreys EB, Mangold LA, Walsh PC. Radical prostatectomy for clinical stage T3a disease. *Cancer.* 2007;109(7):1273–1278.

2. Hsu CY, Wildhagen MF, van Poppel H, Bangma CH. Prognostic factors for and outcome of locally advanced prostate cancer after radical prostatectomy. *BJU Int.* 2010;105(11):1536–1540.

3. Gerber GS, Thisted RA, Chodak GW, et al. Results of radical prostatectomy in men with locally advanced prostate cancer: multi-institutional pooled analysis. *Eur Urol.* 1997;32(4):385–390.

4. Akakura K, Isaka S, Akimoto S, et al. Long-term results of a randomized trial for the treatment of stages B2 and C prostate cancer: radical prostatectomy versus external beam radiation therapy with a common endocrine therapy in both modalities. *Urology.* 1999;54(2):313–318.

Chapter 22

1. Roach M III, Bae K, Speight J, et al. Short-term neoadjuvant androgen deprivation therapy and external-beam radiotherapy for locally advanced prostate cancer: long-term results of RTOG 8610. *J Clin Oncol.* 2008;26(4):585–591.

2. Pilepich MV, Winter K, Lawton CA, et al. Androgen suppression adjuvant to definitive radiotherapy in prostate carcinoma—long-term results of phase III RTOG 85–31. *Int J Radiat Oncol Biol Phys.* 2005;61(5):1285–1290.

3. Bolla M, Gonzalez D, Warde P, et al. Improved survival in patients with locally advanced prostate cancer treated with radiotherapy and goserelin. *N Engl J Med.* 1997;337(5):295–300.

Chapter 23

1. Medical Research Council Prostate Cancer Working Party. Immediate versus deferred treatment for advanced prostatic cancer: initial results of the medical research council trial. *Br J Urol.* 1997;79(2):235–246.

Chapter 25

1. Oefelein MG, Feng A, Scolieri MJ, Ricchiutti D, Resnick MI. Reassessment of the definition of castrate levels of testosterone: implications for clinical decision making. *Urology.* 2000;56(6):1021–1024.

2. Loprinzi CL, Michalak JC, Quella SK, et al. Megestrol acetate for the prevention of hot flashes. *N Engl J Med.* 1994;331(6):347–352.

3. Segal RJ, Reid RD, Courneya KS, et al. Resistance exercise in men receiving androgen deprivation therapy for prostate cancer. *J Clin Oncol.* 2003; 21(9):1653–1659.

4. Perachino M, Cavalli V, Bravi F. Testosterone levels in patients with metastatic prostate cancer treated with luteinizing hormone-releasing hormone therapy: prognostic significance? *BJU Int.* 2010;105(5): 648–651.

5. Salminen EK, Portin RI, Koskinen A, Helenius H, Nurmi M. Associations between serum testosterone fall and cognitive function in prostate cancer patients. *Clin Cancer Res.* 2004;10(22):7575–7582.

6. Tombal B. Appropriate castration with luteinizing hormone-releasing hormone (LHRH) agonists: what is the optimal level of testosterone? *Eur Urol Suppl.* 2005;4(5):14–19.

7. Kaisary AV, Tyrrell CJ, Peeling WB, Griffiths K. Comparison of LHRH analogue (Zoladex) with orchiectomy in patients with metastatic prostatic carcinoma. *Br J Urol.* 1991;67(5):502–508.

Chapter 26

1. Ornstein DK, Rao GS, Johnson B, Charlton ET, Andriole GL. Combined finasteride and flutamide therapy in men with advanced prostate cancer. *Urology.* 1996;48(6):901–905.

2. Crawford ED, Eisenberger MA, McLeod DG, et al. A controlled trial of leuprolide with and without flutamide in prostatic carcinoma. *N Engl J Med.* 1989;321(7):419–424.

3. Leibowitz RL, Tucker SJ. Treatment of localized prostate cancer with intermittent triple androgen blockade: preliminary results in 110 consecutive patients. *Oncologist.* 2001;6(2):177–182.

4. Eisenberger MA, Blumenstein BA, Crawford ED, et al. Bilateral orchiectomy with or without flutamide for metastatic prostate cancer. *N Engl J Med.* 1998;339(15):1036–1042.

Chapter 27

1. Tindall DJ, Rittmaster RS. The rationale for inhibiting 5α-reductase isoenzymes in the prevention and treatment of prostate cancer. *J Urol.* 2008;179(4):1235–1242.

2. Presti JC Jr, Fair WR, Andriole G, et al. Multicenter, randomized, double-blind, placebo-controlled study to investigate the effect of finasteride (MK-906) on stage D prostate cancer. *J Urol.* 1992;148(4):1201–1204.

3. Hedlund PO, Henriksson P. Parenteral estrogen versus total androgen ablation in the treatment of advanced prostate carcinoma: effects on overall survival and cardiovascular mortality. The Scandinavian Prostatic Cancer Group (SPCG)-5 Trial Study. *Urology.* 2000;55(3):328–333.

Chapter 28

1. Kantoff PW, Higano CS, Shore ND, et al. Sipuleucel-T immunotherapy for castration-resistant prostate cancer. *N Eng J Med.* 2010;363(5):411–422.

2. Higano CS, Schellhammer PF, Small EJ, et al. Integrated data from 2 randomized, double-blind, placebo-controlled, phase 3 trials of active cellular immunotherapy with sipuleucel-T in advanced prostate cancer. *Cancer.* 2009;115(16):3670–3679.

Chapter 29

1. Petrylak DP, Tangen CM, Hussain MH, et al. Docetaxel and estramustine compared with mitoxantrone and prednisone for advanced refractory prostate cancer. N Engl J Med. 2004;351(15):1513–1520.

2. Tannock IF, Osoba D, Stockler MR, et al. Chemotherapy with mitoxantrone plus prednisone or prednisone alone for symptomatic hormone-resistant prostate cancer: a Canadian randomized trial with palliative end points. J Clin Oncol. 1996;14(6):1756–1764.

3. Ernst DS, Tannock IF, Winquist EW, et al. Randomized, double-blind, controlled trial of mitoxantrone/prednisone and clodronate versus mitoxantrone/prednisone and placebo in patients with hormone-refractory prostate cancer and pain. J Clin Oncol. 2003;21(17):3335–3342.

4. Kantoff PW, Halabi S, Conaway M, et al. Hydrocortisone with or without mitoxantrone in men with hormone-refractory prostate cancer: results of the cancer and leukemia group B 9182 study. J Clin Oncol. 1999;17(8):2506–2513.

5. Tannock IF, de Wit R, Berry WR, et al. Docetaxel plus prednisone or mitoxantrone plus prednisone for advanced prostate cancer. N Engl J Med. 2004;351(15):1502–1512.

6. A. O. Sartor, S. Oudard, M. Ozguroglu et al. Cabazitaxel or mitoxantrone with prednisone in patients with metastatic castration-resistant prostate cancer (mCRPC) previously treated with docetaxel: final results of a multinational phase III trial (TROPIC). ASCO 2010.

Chapter 30

1. Paes FM, Serafini AN. Systemic metabolic radiopharmaceutical therapy in the treatment of metastatic bone pain. Semin Nucl Med. 2010;40(2):89–104.

2. Saad F, Gleason DM, Murray R, et al. A randomized, placebo-controlled trial of zoledronic acid in patients with hormone-refractory metastatic prostate carcinoma. J Natl Cancer Inst. 2002;94(19):1458–1468.

3. Bamias A, Kastritis E, Bamia C, et al. Osteonecrosis of the jaw in cancer after treatment with bisphosphonates: incidence and risk factors. J Clin Oncol. 2005;23(34):8580–8587.

Chapter 31

1. US National Institutes of Health National Web site: Available at: www .clinicaltrials.gov. Accessed October 2010.

Chapter 33

1. Chan JM, Elkin EP, Silva SJ, Broering JM, Latini DM, Carroll PR. Total and specific complementary and alternative medicine use in a large cohort of men with prostate cancer. Urology. 2005;66(6):1223–1228.

2. Perabo FG, von Low EC, Ellinger J, von Rücker A, Müller SC, Bastian PJ. Soy isoflavone genistein in prevention and treatment of prostate cancer. Prostate Cancer Prostatic Dis. 2008;11:6–12.

3. Sonn GA, Aronson W, Litwin MS. Impact of diet on prostate cancer: a review. Prostate Cancer Prostatic Dis. 2005;8(4):304–310.

Chapter 36

1. Peters L, Sellick K. Quality-of-life of cancer patients receiving inpatient and home-based palliative care. J Adv Nurs. 2006;53(5):524–533.

Index

Note: Throughout the Index, the abbreviation AIPC is used for androgen-independent prostate cancer; AUA for American Urological Association; CAT scan for computed axial tomography scan; DES for diethylstilbestrol; FDA for Food and Drug Administration; GnRH for Gonadotropin-releasing hormone; HIFU for high-intensity focused ultrasound; LHRH for luteinizing hormone-releasing hormone; PSA for prostate-specific antigen; SELECT for Selenium and Vitamin E Cancer Prevention Trial and TURP for transurethral resection of the prostate. Page numbers followed by t indicate tables.

369